SLEEP
REIMAGINED

SLEEP
REIMAGINED

The Fast Track
to a Revitalized Life

DR. PEDRAM NAVAB, FAASM

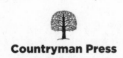

Countryman Press

An Imprint of W. W. Norton & Company
Celebrating a Century of Independent Publishing

This book is intended as a general information resource for people who are having trouble sleeping. It is not a substitute for professional advice. Everyone is different, and no recommendation in this book is intended to substitute for individualized care or any prescribed medication. Anyone who is sleeping less than 6 hours a night and who has been diagnosed with epilepsy or bipolar disorder, is at high risk for falls, or has parasomnias should not try the sleep restriction exercises described in Part II, Session 2. All patients depicted in this book are fictional and all cases described are composites of multiple cases and/or circumstances that typically appear in the patients who are treated for insomnia. Any resemblance between any name, person, situation, or event mentioned or depicted in the book and any actual person, group, situation, or event is coincidental.

For information about permission to reproduce selections from this book, write to Permissions, Countryman Press, 500 Fifth Avenue, New York, NY 10110

For information about special discounts for bulk purchases, please contact W. W. Norton Special Sales at specialsales@wwnorton.com or 800-233-4830

Manufacturing by Lake Book Manufacturing
Production manager: Devon Zahn

Countryman Press
www.countrymanpress.com

An imprint of W. W. Norton & Company, Inc.
500 Fifth Avenue, New York, NY 10110
www.wwnorton.com

978-1-68268-711-6

10 9 8 7 6 5 4 3 2 1

For Stephen N. Brooks, Rafael Pelayo, and
Anstella D. Robinson, for mentoring me during
my early years at Stanford and showing me the
cool side of sleep medicine.

When I let go of what I am, I become what I might be.

—LAO TZU

We don't see things as they are, we see them as we are.

—ANAÏS NIN

There is between sleep and us something like a pact, a treaty with no secret clauses . . .

—MAURICE BLANCHOT

Contents

Contents

Part II
Cognitive Behavioral Therapy for Insomnia (CBT-I)

Introduction

THROUGHOUT MY 16 YEARS AS A SLEEP MEDICINE specialist, this is what I've learned: For your sleep (and life, depending on whom you ask) to fall apart, it doesn't matter if you were just married, discharged from the hospital, won the lottery, or diagnosed with a serious illness. Insomnia can happen in an instant. It can develop gradually. It can even be innate and exert its influence on you as a child. It can happen in the best or worst circumstances, whether you're rich or poor, whether you're living in an opulent home or a tiny apartment. Poor sleep doesn't discriminate. It can happen to the best of us.

All of us have experienced at least one night of abysmal sleep. Conservative estimates reveal that 10% to 30% of adults live with chronic insomnia. Whatever the percentage, it is evident that this is a problem for many of us, and a chronic one at that. Rest assured, though, I have an optimistic outlook, and I believe that even the worst sleep can be reversed. It may not be easy, and it may take some time, but it will improve. It is with this aim that I undertook to write this book: to share the wisdom that I have gleaned from the tens of thousands of patients I've treated over my years of practicing sleep medicine. But it is more than that. It is also a philosophy of sleep, an outlook that not only applies to sleep but also to the various aspects of our lives. Sleep is a continuum, and what you experience in sleep will also segue to your waking life, for good or bad. When individuals sleep better, then hopefulness extends to their waking lives, as well. They feel more in control, and control is power—power to change and power to not allow obstacles to hinder their goals.

The impetus for this book, then, was to attempt to offer treatment to the millions of people who suffer from poor sleep in a practical, entertaining, and easy-to-understand format, whether this poor sleep is characterized as insomnia, a circadian-rhythm disorder, sleep-disordered breathing, or something else. (We'll get to all these conditions later in the corresponding chapters.) Although there is a myriad of sleep disorders in what is considered the diagnostic bible of sleep medicine, *The International Classification of Sleep Disorders*—everything from parasomnias to sleep-related eating disorder to sex-somnia to restless-leg syndrome—this book is designed for those individuals with insomnia or its great imitators. After all, insomnia is the most common sleep disorder, and, as such, will take precedence in this book. Next to sleep-disordered breathing, which we'll discuss in Chapter 6, insomnia is the most common diagnosis I continue to evaluate at my sleep clinic. And it is the most distressing because it is felt more palpably than the rest—a living hell or a zombie nightmare, as most of my patients describe it.

In writing this book, I was reminded of the title of the French electronic-music project M83's album, *Hurry Up, We're Dreaming*. This book is in fact not about dreaming, although the title of the album can extend to sleep insofar as we're all concerned about sleeping: sleeping faster, sleeping more, and sleeping better. This book is all about sleep—specifically, poor sleep that can be improved. But the title of the album is appropriate for our purposes to emphasize that sleep can't be "hurried"; it takes its time, and if you attempt to "hurry sleep," it can actually slow down and exert its stubbornness. Performance anxiety can set in, and insomnia can take over in a most monstrous fashion. Sleep is a natural process, and to exert external pressures on it will simply backfire, as we may have all learned first-hand throughout the years. Rest assured that the techniques we'll use in this book will place some "pressure" on sleep, but it's pressure that is innate and not external or foreign to the system. We may have heard the saying "pressure makes diamonds," but in sleep, being under such pressure will not demonstrate its restorative potential; rather, it will show its destructive potential. Sure, we may have to work to fine-tune our sleep, but it should never resemble real work. Real work does not beget good sleep; in fact, "working at" sleep is anathema to getting good sleep. In this book we'll return to this concept, again and again.

I continue to remember the ending sequence of the great American drama series *The Waltons*, which aired from 1972 to 1981. I was a child then, but I still remember the lines at the end of each episode when everyone appeared to go to bed at the same time each night and say their goodnights. The sequence would sound like this: Elizabeth: "Good night, John Boy." John Boy: "Good night, Elizabeth. Good night, Daddy," and so on and so forth until every one of the parents, grandparents, and 7 kids had said their goodnights.

During my training as a sleep specialist, I would always reflect on how inaccurate this depiction was, that sleep was not this artificial or imposed. No one family could make its members sleep at the same time, no matter how hard they tried. In fact, the harder one tries to sleep, the less successful they will be. But to see this scene played over and over again for almost a decade reinforced in me the notion that sleep should be uniform, that everyone *could* sleep at the same time each and every night. (As a child, when I couldn't sleep, I would always blame myself. I thought that I somehow wasn't doing something "right," that something was wrong with me. As a sleep expert, I now know better.)

But sleep is not uniform. It is different things for different people. For insomniacs, it is a chore or "dread," as most have come to call their albatross. Most insomniacs treat their bed as a painful bed of nails because that is how *psychologically* uncomfortable it is for them. They are overstimulated when they attempt to unsuccessfully sleep in their beds. We'll tackle this issue with our first case, Laura, who loathed her bed after a traumatic incident but was drawn to it like an opium fiend.

This book is a little different from most sleep books. Sure, it will cover the essentials of what one needs to know about sleep and how to treat insomnia and its imitators. It will show you how to think about sleep so that it doesn't feel like a category of its own, separate from one's waking life. But it is also a book of narratives, a literary book of sorts, based on the actual experiences of patients whom I've seen over the years that exemplify the various sleep conditions at their most elemental. These stories are distilled to the conditions that patients of mine actually experienced, so that readers can identify with the sleep disturbances and the treatments that real people successfully underwent. Each story is rooted in patterns and symptoms that I have witnessed in my patients throughout the years. I undertook to write these stories to make it easier for you to recognize and relate the sleep concepts I discuss in a concrete and personal way.

This book is similar to the books written by British neurologist and author Oliver Sacks in which he recounts his patients' bizarre histories in order to better understand the pathologies that cause their neurological oddities. However, this book differs in certain aspects from Sacks'. First, unlike Sacks' stories that address the oddities—the "zebras," if you will—this book is about the common "horses," the different types of insomnia that the sleep-medicine specialist is exposed to on a daily basis. Second, Sacks does not offer explanations of treatment. Unlike Sacks, I intend to fully address treatment for the particular patient and immerse you, the reader, in that history. After all, this book is about treating your insomnia, not just depicting it. The individual stories are a starting point, to anchor the symptoms, so that you, as readers, can relate and understand the psychology of why you might be experiencing your symptoms. After all, we're here to diagnose and treat your insomnia.

At the Stanford Sleep Disorders Clinic, where I was a fellow, we had developed a cognitive behavioral therapy program for insomnia with two clinical psychologists. The sessions comprised six participants who, in a group setting, discussed the specific issues with their inability to sleep well. We clinicians were there to assist them and develop a plan for each, in a collaborative milieu. It may sound counterintuitive, but the sessions worked, even if these individuals had different sets of concerns and issues regarding their insomnia. These workshops were excellent in allowing others to understand that they were not alone, that other participants had concerns and symptoms just like them. It created a unique bond between the participants, in which they felt powerful and in control of exorcising their sleep demons. They listened to each other's stories. Through these narratives, they not only learned about one another but were also able to place themselves in the other's situation. This is what this book aims to do through its stories.

A bit about the construction of this book: it is really two books in one. The first part comprises narratives to reinforce sleep concepts. The second portion begins to explain the process of cognitive behavioral therapy for insomnia (CBT-I), which is the foundation for treating insomnia without medications. Thus, one may approach this text in a myriad of ways. One way is to get the lay of the land, delving into some of the stories first and reviewing the first few weeks of CBT-I. Or, one can read the entirety of the second part of the book first and then read the narratives to reinforce the concepts of CBT-I. Whichever way you choose to read this book will be fine.

I hope that with this book you feel you have a comfortable environment—a safe space, if you will—to examine sleep in all its goodness and badness. The individual profiles are there to illustrate specific sleep issues you might experience most nights or every night. The second part of the book, then, will introduce you to sleep concepts and reinforce what you have learned from the narratives.

In Part 1, we'll present stories of people who have difficulties with their sleep. You may relate to the people I'm calling Laura, Stephen, or Jeremy, struggling to sleep after traumatic life events. You might be like Savannah, Bruce, or Mary, whose sleep is disrupted by their schedules. Your anxiety about sleep may resemble Ava's, who continually ruminates about unforeseen consequences that her insomnia could cause. Or, you might find you are like Allen and Thao, whose insomnia stems from medical conditions that have not been diagnosed. No matter your circumstance, as the diversity of these individual stories would suggest, there are many sleep disorders. But there are also many ways we can respond to and try to improve our sleep. Relating our sleep situations to those of individual people described in these chapters may make us feel less alone than we thought.

Sleep will fall apart for everyone at some point—maybe for a night, maybe for years. That is a given, based on the statistics we have. However, fortunately, sleep can be restored and maintained. I'm hopeful that these narratives will help you to understand that to be asleep is not so different from the simplicity of being awake. In fact, our brain-wave activity during a certain portion of sleep—REM sleep—is quite similar to wakefulness. Through these stories, and through description of my CBT-I practice, we can explore just how that restoration process can look for you. Ultimately, I hope you will walk away from this book with a clear road map to new and improved sleep—sleep reimagined.

SLEEP
REIMAGINED

PART I

THE CASE STUDIES

Case 1

Laura

Psychophysiological Insomnia
and Sleep Restriction

I MET LAURA, A 42-YEAR-OLD ADVERTISING EXECUTIVE, on a very hot August afternoon in my West Los Angeles exam room. We were in a recently-cemented COVID-19 world, with Laura sporting a basic black mask tightly wrapped around her nose and mouth as well as a black baseball cap, a tuft of blonde hair escaping from the opening in the back. She arrived looking heartbroken, as if she had just emerged from a failed relationship. Her dazzling blue eyes shone, although I could recognize that they were brighter and stronger before this pandemic that had stolen the person she once was. She had had difficulty finding metered parking in the busy streets and, as a result, had been 15 minutes late to our appointment. I opened the door and she quickly initiated the conversation.

"Sorry for being so late."

"No problem. We live in the craziness of Los Angeles and now this pandemic, don't we?"

"Yes, we do. But thanks for being so understanding. It's just that with this COVID nightmare everything feels so abnormal now. I can't stand it."

"It's not easy for anyone. That's for sure."

"Thanks again for being so considerate. Do you mind if I wear my sunglasses? The light irritates my eyes."

She searched distractedly for the reflective Ray-Ban aviator sunglasses in her purse, finally found them, and put them on. I saw myself in her artificial eyes but couldn't *see* her. She was somewhere else. She was so reticent that I realized coming to see a sleep doctor was probably a difficult decision for her.

"So, what can I do for you, Ms. Cavallari?"

"Please call me Laura. I prefer it that way."

"Okay, Laura. What seems to be the issue?"

She looked away from me for a few seconds, before her glasses met my eyes.

"Well, I contracted coronavirus in early June and was in the hospital for a week. I had a high fever and problems breathing, and so I was told by my family doctor to go to the hospital. I'm glad I did, because a few days later I had to be placed on steroids and on an antiviral cocktail. I felt that I was suffocating. I couldn't get air in my lungs."

"I'm sorry to hear that. It must have been so difficult for you."

"Thanks. It was. But I somehow got through it. I'm thankful that I'm alive. It was such a harrowing experience that I'd never like to relive."

Now she looked at the linoleum floor, her hands clasped. Her knuckles were stretched taut. She rocked in her chair a bit before she started speaking again.

"But, you know, I had the best sleep before all this, and now my sleep has gone to shit, to utter shit. . . . Sorry. I didn't mean to curse, but I'm such a mess now."

Whereas her tone and rhythm were slow and monotonous before, their volume and tempo had suddenly increased, as if this was a truth she couldn't suppress any longer. Now her words came faster, the pitch of her voice rising correspondingly.

"I mean, I had the best sleep before I contracted this virus, and when I went to the hospital, my sleep fell apart. But now that I'm, for the most part, back to my baseline health, my sleep has remained the same as when I contracted the virus."

"What was your situation like at the hospital?"

"I've never been hospitalized before, so it was a strange environment. And, to add to it, my boyfriend couldn't visit me. That was distressing on another level. But every day I was surrounded by bright lights, nurses taking my blood, being woken up to eat, and so on. I couldn't stand it. And forget about sleep. I don't think I got any while I was there."

"How many hours would you say you slept each night before your hospitalization?"

"Eight hours, easy. I fell asleep almost instantaneously every night at 11 p.m., never woke up throughout the night, and got out of bed at 7 a.m. to start my day. My boyfriend, who sometimes sleeps over in the same bed as I do, would envy me. Between the two of us, he was the insomniac. I was begrudged."

She smiled a bit when she said this and then returned to her sullen expression.

"So, you had great sleep, then poor sleep when you went to the hospital, and what happened when you returned home?"

"I thought my insomnia would resolve because I didn't have to deal with distracting and annoying things in the hospital, but I just lay there and couldn't go to sleep. It was, and continues to be, a disaster."

I explained to Laura that she was experiencing what we call psychophysiological insomnia. This type of insomnia results in tension and learned sleep-preventing associations, creating decreased functioning during wakefulness. In other words, when she was exposed to stimuli in the hospital—the lights, the beeps, the constant vigilance of nurses—she had developed insomnia. And although she had returned to her normal environment, that initial insomnia she had experienced while she was in the hospital had now created its own new insomnia. Her concern then was about the lack of sleep she had gotten at the hospital. She was now constantly ruminating about getting a "good night's sleep" because her poor sleep was now the culprit, not the stimuli at the hospital. Her insomnia was now motivated by the insomnia itself.

"I never thought about it that way, but you're right. I can't stop thinking about the fact that I can't go to sleep. I'm always thinking about getting the sleep that I had before this illness. It truly dictates everything in my life right now."

"Exactly. But do you see the issue before us?"

"Sort of. I try to just lie in bed, thinking that I may catch some sleep if I'm there long enough. But it doesn't happen. And then, before I know it, the sun has risen, and I have to start my day, feeling extremely groggy and sleepy throughout the day."

Laura took off her sunglasses briefly to show the dark circles underneath her eyes and then replaced the sunglasses just as quickly.

"I'm so ashamed of these circles. The light hurts my eyes, too, but the circles are the reasons that I wear my sunglasses inside. I wasn't completely honest with you before."

"It's perfectly fine. No judgments here. So, do you just lie in bed? For how long?"

"Well, I go to bed at 9 p.m., thinking that I can get more sleep if I go to bed earlier, but nothing happens until at least midnight, when I doze off slightly. Then I wake up about 2 hours later and can't return to sleep for at least another hour. I finally wake up at 7 a.m., feeling groggy as hell. In total, I'm getting about 6 hours of sleep, but it's so broken up and erratic. I can't function this way."

"I got you. There are two issues here. One is stimulus control, meaning that you have paired the concept of the bed with not being able to sleep. That's a conditioned response because the bed is not a place of repose for you anymore. It is now associated with poor sleep and your history at the hospital. In other words, your normal cues about sleep—rest, being energized in the morning after a good night's sleep, and so forth—are now paired more frequently with responses other than sleep. Do you see that?"

"Yeah, I think so. I no longer see my bed as a restful space. I dread sleeping there every night because I know that it will make me even more tired the following day."

"Exactly. Our objective for you, then, is to dissociate your bed with unrest and associate it again with sleep. That means you will have to get out of bed every time you can't sleep, so that your bed is not associated with your inability to sleep. That is the concept of stimulus control therapy."

Although I still couldn't see Laura's eyes, I could see that her lips were less sullen now and that they were becoming more inquisitive, as if she was eager to ask a question.

"So, I should really be getting out of bed every time I can't sleep? How cruel!"

"It is a bit cruel, I guess, but we need to make the association between your bedroom environment very robust and clear. Boundaries between your bed and the rest of your home are necessary if we are to create a robust link between your bed and sleep. If you can't fall asleep within 30 minutes, get out of bed, go to the living room, look through a magazine, keep the lights dim, and return to bed when you feel slightly sleepy. Don't use the computer, read a book, or anything stimulating. You must also set boundaries between this 'media stimulation,' as I like to call it, and your sleep. These things will awaken your brain and serve as reminders of what is going on in your life and the world."

"Don't I know it! The news these days makes me feel so hellishly anxious and fearful. So, I keep getting out of bed every time I can't fall asleep within 30 minutes?"

"Yes, exactly."

"I have done this a couple of times, and sometimes I have fallen asleep on the couch."

"Well, that was a lost opportunity, because if you had gone to bed then, you would have paired your sleepiness with your bed and the bedroom environment, which is exactly what we want."

"Let me ask you this. What if I start to get energized again once I start to head to my bed? What do I do then?"

"I think you know the answer to that question."

"Seriously? You'd want me to return to the living room again until I feel sleepy again?"

"Yes. I know it's tough, and it will be for the first few weeks or so, but that is the only way we can associate your bed with sleep. Now, there is one other concept that I'd like to go over before we end this session.

This is probably the most important concept that we'll use for you. It's called sleep restriction."

"That doesn't sound very appealing. Does that mean you want me to sleep less?"

Laura smirked at this statement, but I could tell that she had felt a blow after she had been offered a way out of her misery. She now looked despondently at me. She continued.

"How does that work, exactly?"

"I'm afraid that it kind of works like it sounds. You say that you go to bed at 9 p.m. because you're trying to maximize your sleep, but despite that, you're only getting 6 hours of sleep. From what you said to me before, you're in bed from 9 p.m. to 7 a.m., which is total of 10 hours, and only 6 hours of that are spent asleep. Do you see how inefficient that is?"

"When you put it that way, I guess it's not great."

She doffed her sunglasses then and looked directly at me as if she had embarked upon an understanding that she had previously been deprived of.

"What do you propose that I do, then? Go to bed later?"

"Yes, you hit the concept on its head. So, if you're not sleeping until at least midnight, then go to bed at that time. Initially, you will come to loath me because you're probably going to get less than your 6 hours. I get it, and some of my patients give up at that point. That's expected because you will still probably have insomnia at midnight. But what we're achieving is great in the long run. As you get more tired that week, your homeostatic drive to sleep, meaning your increased tendency to sleep because of the deprivation, will become stronger and stronger, and you will naturally fall asleep. More importantly, you will also have relinked that association between sleep and bed, which you previously had, before your hospitalization. Does that make sense?"

"Yes, it does. I would get up at the same time?"

"Absolutely. No matter what time you fall asleep, you must get up at the same time. That will strengthen your natural circadian rhythms and prime your body for sleep throughout the day. Your get-up time is your anchor. You can't sleep in past that time. As I previously said, you will feel sleepier during this initial period, but that's what we want—for the sleep drive to get stronger and stronger. You'll have to stick to this schedule on both weekdays and weekends, until we normalize your sleep."

"Okay, I see that. Do I need to do anything else?"

"Yes, please keep a sleep diary and write the number of hours of sleep you're getting each night for that week. Average the number of hours of sleep that you're getting and divide that by the number of hours that you're in bed. That number is our sleep efficiency. If your sleep efficiency is less than 80%, then we need to actually have you go to bed later, and if it's more than 85%, we can have you to go to bed earlier. If your sleep efficiency is between 80% to 85%, we can keep your schedule the same. You're rewarded with more time in bed—and, hopefully, sleep—if your sleep efficiency is higher."

I could tell that Laura was calculating not the number of hours that she'd be getting but rather how sleep-deprived she would be. She was now looking at the linoleum floor again, somehow dispirited that I had brought this concept of sleep restriction to the table. She started speaking again.

"Can I just focus on the other therapy—the stimulus therapy, I think you said—and forget about this concept of sleep deprivation?"

There was an involuntary sly grin on my face because this concept had nothing to do with sleep deprivation. I wasn't a monster after all, but at this point in therapy, patients thought I was absolutely insane. They had come into the sleep clinic to get more sleep, and I was telling them to sleep less.

"It's not actually sleep deprivation but rather sleep restriction. It's easy to confuse the two. But you must try to implement both concepts simultaneously. Okay?"

"Yeah, I guess that's fine. I don't know how successful I'll be, but I'll try."

"Let's stop here for today because I don't want to throw a lot of concepts at you during the first session. I'd prefer that you learn a couple of concepts well than know a little about everything. How does that sound?"

"I like that idea. Is there anything I should do for our next session?"

"Yes. As I previously mentioned, I'm going to ask you to keep a sleep diary, jotting down your impressions of your sleep at night for about 5 nights. It doesn't have to be detailed, but I just want to gauge how you slept, how you felt when you woke up, and the number of hours of sleep you obtained for that night. And, of course, calculating the average of your sleep efficiency for that week. It shouldn't be a difficult task. Are you up for the challenge?"

"I've battled this damn virus, so I think I can do this. Apologies, again. My insomnia brings out the worst in me."

"No worries. I'll see you next week, then. We need to have close follow-ups during the initial sessions, and as your sleep improves, we can lengthen the interim between sessions. By the way, I want you to be honest in your journal. All I care about is your sleep efficiency and your bedtime routine. Otherwise, you can keep the diary to yourself and make it a part of your general well-being, detailing other events in your life. I think that will also be good for you in other aspects."

I could tell that the shimmer of hope had returned to her eyes. Laura walked resolutely out of the office as if she were determined to make her sleep better. I imagined the Los Angeles heat enveloping her, as she walked to her car, turned on the ignition, and headed home to Santa Monica just as the blistering sun was about to set.

LAURA'S SLEEP DIARY
August 15, 2020

I felt super-excited about tackling my insomnia after seeing the doctor yesterday. Despite what he told me, I went to bed at 9 p.m. last night. I'm trying to give myself a couple of days before I tackle this sleep-deprivation thing. I know the doctor won't like this. I couldn't fall asleep. Again. Todd wanted to come over, but I made up some excuse of having a migraine. He's really cross with me these days, although he understands that I battled a pretty brutal illness. I don't really want him to know that I was so desperate as to see a doctor. Not that he'd really care and not that there's anything wrong with this, but I want to keep this to myself for now and appear stronger than I actually am. I was so independent before contracting this coronavirus and I don't want this to change his perception of me. I finally slept at midnight, feeling a little groggy, but, wouldn't you know it, just like clockwork, I woke up a couple of hours later. However, instead of lying there, I went to the living room and browsed through an old issue of Vogue. Looking at those beautiful models depressed me (especially because I feel and look terrible now, having lost some hair from the illness), and I immediately felt a little groggy. I threw that magazine in the trash can. I didn't need to see those unrealistic models again. I went to bed 15 minutes later (instead of my usual hour) and, surprisingly, didn't wake up until 7 a.m. This morning, I don't feel great, but I also don't feel as bad as I did the night before. Baby steps, I tell myself, baby steps. That's how things are done.

August 16, 2020

It was so hot last night, but I turned the air conditioner way up and was able to bring some semblance of normalcy back to the apartment. I can't take this COVID-19 business anymore. Everywhere I look, there it is. More people are dying every day, so I'm trying to see less and less television these days and read the newspaper less. I need to concentrate on my health. That's the important thing. After I returned from work, I cooked dinner—some pasta and store-bought sauce. It tasted okay, but I'm not into food these days. I've probably lost at least 10 pounds between the hospital and now. Todd didn't call last night. He probably realizes I need some space. I appreciate and love him. I hope he realizes this. At 9 p.m.,

I was wide awake. I contemplated whether I should go to bed, but I decided to take the doctor's advice and stay up until midnight. This is new to me. I wouldn't have had the courage before. This is a good sign. It's been a while since I slept at midnight. I was a bit frightened by the prospect of getting less sleep. Thinking about this sleep deprivation thing sickens me. But I'll try to follow the good doctor's advice. I hope he's right. Well, I definitely felt sleepy at 11:30 p.m. but decided to stay up for another 30 minutes and follow his exact regimen. But wouldn't you know it? As soon as my head hit the pillow at midnight, I was suddenly awake again, thinking that this is going to be another bad night. It took me about an hour to fall asleep. I fell asleep at 1 a.m. and then awoke at 3 a.m. I went to the living room and leafed through Architectural Digest *this time. I couldn't stand seeing those models again, with their perfect bodies and faces. Fifteen minutes later, I was super tired and went to bed, sleeping until 7 a.m. The doctor had told me not to sleep past 7 a.m., so I didn't. I woke up, probably feeling more tired than I ever had. I calculated my hours of sleep and it was 5.5 hours, instead of my usual 6. I was on the path to sleep deprivation. I would give this another 3 days, but if this is how it will be, I won't continue. I usually don't give up so easily, but this insomnia has really devastated me.*

August 17, 2020

Have I turned the corner? Last night was much better. I left work at 5 p.m., headed from Downtown LA to Santa Monica. Surprisingly, there was little traffic and I was home within 30 minutes. I cooked pasta again (the only food I can manage to make), ate some fruit, and watched Ozark *on Netflix. I need to get my mind off this virus. I called Todd afterwards and told him my situation, how much I missed him, and how I'd like to see him this weekend. He told me that he missed me, too, and agreed that we should meet. We planned to do some hiking at Runyon Canyon Park this weekend. If there was a large crowd, we planned on ditching that and going elsewhere. I realize that I'm probably not infectious anymore, but I want to take as much precautions as I can. I don't want some poor person contracting this awful disease from me. I spent the remainder of the night paying late bills on the computer and doing laundry. It was exhausting, but I did it. It was already 11 p.m., and I decided to give this sleep deprivation, or sleep restriction thing, another chance. I know the doctor had told me this was a difficult week, so I thought I should give it a decent attempt. I went to bed at midnight and fell asleep at 12:30 a.m. I couldn't believe it. This was a first for me since being hospitalized. I woke up at 3 a.m., but then fell asleep within a few minutes. I didn't even have to go to the living room this time. I woke up at 7 a.m., feeling kind of refreshed, if you can believe that! In total, I got about 6.5 hours of sleep, but was only in bed for 7 hours. The doctor will be so proud of me. I may actually have a chance at this! "May" is the operative word here. I'm cautiously optimistic.*

August 18, 2020

I may have been a little overconfident based on my sleep last night. But let's start with the day after my "good" sleep. I had immediately felt more energized than I ever had since my hospitalization. Cherise even noticed my energy when I came to work. "Wow, you look so rested," she said. "What did you do?" I lied to her, telling her that I had gone on a great date the previous night. It's so sad that I have to fabricate, but I just don't want people to know that I'm an insomniac. I don't know why I have such a taboo about it. Millions of people suffer from this condition, and here I am, wallowing in my grief. "So, Todd, huh?" she said. "Well, everyone enjoys a late night now and then, right?" I laughed it off and went back to work. I hate lying to Cherise, because she's such a good friend, but I have no choice. I don't want her to know my secret. I left work, picked up some deli concoction at Whole Foods, and headed straight to the apartment. I think that Ms. Grigoryan even noticed the spring in my step. "Glad you're feeling better, dear," she said, not recognizing that she had given herself away from what she had not said the other day. "I am, thank you," I responded. I have to stop thinking, or over thinking, about things so critically. I ate dinner, spoke to Todd about our outing this weekend, and caught up on some work for the ad campaign that our agency is running. Before I knew it, it was midnight and I was excited again to sleep. But this time, I was just lying there again, like I had the nights before. Last night was a fluke, then, I told myself. God damn it! I couldn't believe it. It took me about an hour to fall asleep and then I woke up at 3 a.m., heading for the living room at 3:30 a.m. before retiring to bed at 3:45 a.m. I slept until 7 a.m., when the alarm clock went off so belligerently. I slept about 5 and a half hours, which wasn't horrible, but it was less than the night before. I don't know what to say. Maybe I should just give up on this thing before I give myself hope that will once again evaporate.

August 19, 2020

I'm yo-yoing. I guess that's the only way to describe it. I was a mess again yesterday. I arrived to work late and had to get a latte at this café place, Insomnia Coffee Shop on Beverly and Fair-fax. The perfect name for a coffee place, although I don't want to remind myself of the problems that I already have. I told myself that I wouldn't drink coffee, so I ordered a steamer—oat milk with some vanilla—instead. How low I've gone—no caffeine at a coffee shop—I reminded myself. I actually was on time to work. Cherise *had taken the day off, so I didn't have to explain my wretched state of affairs. I left work as soon as the clock struck 5 p.m. and headed home. I was super tired, but I decided to work some more on our ad campaign. I mistakenly turned on the TV and learned that the worldwide mortality count from COVID-19 was now close to 6 million! The thought depressed me, but I realized how lucky I was. I cursed the president again for his mishandling of this entire situation and decided to turn the television off for good tonight. I ate the leftovers from Whole Foods and watched more Ozark episodes. That show is so addictive. It was almost midnight, and I was dreading another sleepless night. I went to bed and instantly fell asleep. For the first time since I left the hospital, I was able to sleep the entire night! I woke up at 7 a.m., feeling refreshed. It was a strange feeling. Was this me? I wanted to shout this to the world. I did it. This sleep restriction thing had worked. I knew that I would have good and bad nights, but this was a great start. I'll be seeing the doctor on Monday. I can't wait to tell him how my sleep is slowly improving. I know that I'll have bad days here and there, but he said that was expected. My hike with Todd couldn't have come at a better time. I really miss him.*

I saw Laura on the pixelated screen on my telemedicine portal. She instantly smiled at me. Her sunglasses were nowhere in sight. Wearing a white blouse, she adjusted her screen a bit. Her voice was stronger and happier, despite the bad connection and irregular reception. She looked fresh.

"How are you, Laura?"

"Hi, I'm doing much better. Thank you."

"How was your week of sleep deprivation?"

She instantly laughed, her eyes blinking in slow fashion, given the erratic technology. I could see that she was no longer in her old world, where things were chaotic and messy.

"Ha! It's sleep restriction, Doc. Don't you know that?"

"Good. Just trying to test you. Well, let's get to it. How did you do over the last 5 days?

"I'm happy to report that my sleep efficiency for last week was around 85%. I don't have the exact number, but not lying in bed for those extra 3 hours really made the difference. There were nights that are not as good as some really stellar nights, but overall, I am sleeping significantly better than when I first spoke to you. A big thanks to you."

"Good sleep was already in you. You just had to think differently about it. That's all. We all know what to do, but common sense doesn't always win the good fight."

"Well, those techniques worked. I'm actually a lot more optimistic and energetic."

"I can see that. Our problem isn't over yet. Insomnia has a way of rearing its ugly head when you least expect it. Just remember to be steadfast and continue this regimen for at least the next 6 weeks. You don't necessarily need to continue this calculation past that time because it will come naturally. But continue to keep your sleep journal and calculate your sleep efficiency every night. Well, you know what your sleep efficiency tells us, right?"

"I'm confused. What does what mean?"

"Just the fact that you get an extra 15 minutes more in bed because of your stellar sleep efficiency. If your sleep efficiency is greater than 85%, you can go to bed 15 minutes earlier. If it's less than 80%, you actually need to go to bed 15 minutes later. If it's between 80% and 85%, you maintain the same sleep schedule."

"Yay! So, I can go to bed at 11:45 p.m., then?"

"Yep. You deserve it."

"Fantastic!"

"Let's meet again next week via this portal. That will provide us with more data and we'll have to go over some more important concepts related to cognitive behavioral therapy. But you're on the right path, so continue what you've been doing. Also, remember that you should focus on what you can control. There is no use in freezing up when things don't go your way. Use that as an opportunity to work things out and become stronger. Your sleep will be the better for it."

"That's important to remember. Thank you!"

Just as quickly, Laura's image faded from the screen. What lingered, though, and showed, was her tenacity through her ordeal, not only of her infection, but the insomnia that ensued.

☾

Sleep Pearls

The most important takeaway from Laura's story is that she didn't give up on sleep restriction, and this was the real key to her success. Sleep restriction is one of the main tenets of the cognitive behavioral therapy program for insomnia because it is such a powerful concept. Learn and practice this well.

Another important concept here was stimulus control therapy, used in conjunction with sleep restriction, so Laura was able to reset her associations with the bed and bedroom environment. Though it was tempting to pick up those *Vogue* subscriptions, she knew to put away mentally distressing media at the right time. She ditched other stimuli like coffee, and ultimately, she was able to successfully cement and closely realign her sleep with her bed, so that the bed no longer became a signal of her inability to sleep.

Restructuring your ideas about sleep and your attitude toward your sleeping environment may not be easy. As we saw with Laura, it can take time and result in some difficult first days. But just as it was for Laura, reducing stimulation and practicing sleep restriction can be worth it in the end.

Case 2

Ava

Catastrophizing and Performance Anxiety

Dear Carrie,

I'm sleeping less and less each night. I no longer feel "sharp." It's affecting my work as an in-house counsel at the film studio. Although there is a plethora of therapists here (and, believe me, every one of our clients has at least one), I can't seem to get myself to see one. I recognize that I'm depressed. But it's more than that. I'm anxious all the time, especially when I arrive at the law offices located in the studio itself. I'm sure that my insomnia is causing many of my symptoms. I try to make eye contact with the grips, the sound technicians, and the rest of the production team as I walk to the office. They're aloof, in their own world. I smile at them while they walk, but they don't see me. Perhaps I've turned into a ghost now. I can't tell anymore. I don't know if this made-up world has become my new reality. I see costumed actors exiting trailers. Caterers setting up between takes. I see an ersatz western town juxtaposed against the brownstones of Brooklyn and come to realize that this made-up fantasy is what grounds me and my profession as an attorney. But it's not true. It's actually the other way around. My work has never seemed more unreal to me, drafting and negotiating development and production contracts for projects that seem out of my reach, part of some fantasy world I won't ever understand. I'm not making any sense, am I? I often think that, too, as if my mind were somewhere else. If you haven't figured it out already, my sleep hasn't gotten any better since I last wrote to you. I have a feeling that despite my arduous work here and my deserved promotion, my growing carelessness in reviewing the contracts will eventually show itself. The culprit may be my sleepiness. I may get fired. Those are my fears—mediocrity and rejection. After this endless volley with myself, I've finally decided to see a psychiatrist. I held it off for as long as I could. I'm depressed and anxious. I need to be on medication. It's nothing more than a chemical imbalance, I tell myself.

So I made an appointment with a psychiatrist, Dr. Hoyt, and saw her yesterday.

This is how my encounter went with her:

"You're Ava, right? Pleased to meet you. My name is Dr. Hoyt, but please call me Julia. Follow me into my office."

I followed her, this woman who seemed so sure of herself, yet very gentle at the same time. Her perfume was musky and sweet, hard and soft, exactly like the demeanor she exuded.

"What can I do for you?" Julia's tone was aggressive yet gentle, and her manner was blunt.

"Well," I started, "I've felt very down lately. I know that I'm depressed and part of that has to do with my disillusionment with Los Angeles and with my occupation." She paused, but then replied.

"I see. This seems to be really bothering you. You haven't encountered this problem before. I can sense it. You seem a little nervous to me."

Her statement surprised me. Did I look nervous to others? I told her that, yes, this was the first time I had actually felt depressed, and I didn't really want to associate with others. I told her that outside of the office, I had kept to myself. I hadn't really socialized. For the past 6 months, I also hadn't slept more than 5 hours per night, ruminating about my job and whether I would be fired for my carelessness in reviewing contracts. Due to my lack of sleep, I also felt that I would fall asleep behind the wheel."

"Well, that's easy enough to fix. Just quit your job and start a new profession, dear. And stop driving. Just take Uber," she said.

I thought she was joking, but she was dead serious. In some strange way, her suggestions made sense, but they were extreme and unpractical. I actually liked being an attorney. I just couldn't cope with my lack of sleep and the frustration that this brought.

"The next best thing, of course, is medication. Am I right, or what? Medication is the key to all things. A little Xanax here, a little Seroquel. And you mix that in with some Silenor. It's actually like baking a cake. You have access to all the ingredients in the supermarket, and you have to know what to buy and in what quantity. It's actually kind of fun, if you ask me, this experimentation," she continued.

I didn't know what to say. Was she serious? Like baking a cake?

"I guess so. You're the doctor here," I said, hesitating.

She replied instantaneously: "That settles it, then. Here is a prescription for Ambien CR, Zoloft, and Seroquel for your insomnia and depression. We can always add some Silenor and Xanax to the mix down the line. I'll add a bit of Ativan now, in case you feel the nervous bug coming on. You never know when that little monster will rear its head. And of course, we can add more to your regimen once we see how things develop with your medication armamentarium." She sounded like I was going into war, and the medications were my armor and weapons.

"Do you think I need all these medications? I said. "It seems an awful lot. I currently don't take any medications. I barely take Advil unless I'm in a lot of pain."

"It's fine, dear," she replied. "You'll see. Meds are our friends, especially working in Tinseltown. How do you think these celebrities cope? Most are drugged to the core and then some. Trust me. I treat several of them. And they're not doing too badly, am I right? I'll see you in a couple of weeks, dear. We'll see how this is all working out for you. Zoloft and Seroquel will take about 6 weeks to kick in, but you should notice the effects of the rest right away."

Was she trying to drug me into some sort of coma, so I couldn't distinguish reality from fiction? I took the scripts, said my goodbyes, and left the office. I didn't plan on returning.

Lost more than ever,

Ava

Her name was Ava. She was an attorney working in the legal department of a Los Angeles film studio. She was bright and hopeful, although there was a hint of pessimism in her tone that implied she was disappointed with other doctors she'd seen before. Her eyebrows furrowed a bit. Based on what she was saying, she was also depressed and was recently prescribed Zoloft to temper her downcast mood. The glamorous lifestyle that had beckoned her from her hometown in Tucson, Arizona, had been illusory. She felt like the only "real" thing among the fake tapestries and people of the studio world where she worked. Often, she felt like a ghost, traversing the city, overlooked and underappreciated by everyone. She had a best friend, Carrie, with whom she readily communicated via traditional letters. I had asked why she didn't just *talk* to her best friend.

"Because I always express myself so much better through letters, getting the meaning just right, without any interruption or losing my train of thought. I've actually begun to feel, too, that speaking feels abnormal and strange because I hardly speak with anyone anymore. Except when I'm at work," she said. "It's kind of pathetic, really. I feel like I'm just taking pills for the pain and insomnia. I don't even feel like I'm in control anymore."

There was no doubt that she was experiencing a major depressive episode. I didn't need to ask to know that her depressive disorder was probably a culmination of different events throughout her life and, in particular, her move to Los Angeles. I dug a bit further regarding her sleep issues.

"What can I do for your sleep?" I said. "After all, I'm a sleep doctor."

"Well, although I feel less depressed with the use of an antidepressant, my sleep has not improved. I've been taking Zoloft for a total of 6 weeks now, and I may need to take that for a longer period of time. But my sleep is still pretty bad. "

I knew I was dealing with someone who genuinely cared about her health. She was determined to make herself better, even amid this depressive episode. She hadn't given up hope yet.

I suggested that insomnia and depression often coexist together and it's difficult to say what occurred first. Did the insomnia cause the depression or vice versa? Both need to be treated because otherwise it becomes a vicious cycle, both making one another dependent on another and spiraling each out of control. It is an abusive relationship. Ava agreed with that, but she really wanted to work on her sleep. She said that she was recently prescribed Ambien CR but had several episodes where she found food in her bed and realized she had ransacked her kitchen the night before.

"Do you have a history of sleepwalking, or somnambulism, as we like to say?" I asked her.

"Yes, I believe that I had numerous episodes as a child, but I then outgrew them. My parents also had that diagnosis as children."

"Yes, sleepwalking tends to be genetic and run in families. The episodes you had are related to your taking Ambien combined with your history of sleepwalking. The two don't mix well. If you haven't already, discontinue your sleeping medication and we'll start on a course of cognitive behavioral therapy for insomnia."

Ava went on to say that she often found herself in bed thinking about the next day, about how tired she would be and the consequences of that fatigue. She had the feeling that she would be fired from her job for her carelessness in reviewing contracts.

"You know, I feel like I'm this close to being fired. I feel so inattentive sometimes, especially when I'm reviewing my clients' contracts. It's no small feat, and one really has to be vigilant about details."

"Well, let me ask you, have you ever been reprimanded for this, for your carelessness, as you say?"

"No, but I feel like I'm on the verge. You know, each day brings me closer to that inevitable admonition, 'You're this close to being fired.' That's what I fear most."

"Let's untangle that, then, because this seems to be your fear, your 'catastrophizing' of the situation, as we sleep doctors like to call it," I replied.

"Okay. I've actually read about this online when I was researching treatments for insomnia. That means I'm blowing things out of proportion, right?" she said.

"Exactly. There appears to be a mismatch between what you think will happen and the probability of that actually occurring. For example, let's say you have had insomnia for 4 years, which is what you told me. That's about 200 weeks. If you've had insomnia three times per week during that time, then that's about 600 nights when you couldn't sleep. Now, you mentioned that you were fairly certain that you would be fired or get into a car crash after those sleepless nights. So, let's say that's 80% of those occasions. If we calculate those odds, that would be about 480 times of your having been fired or gotten into a car accident. Now, how many times have you actually been fired or involved in a car accident?" I said.

She hesitated a bit before answering. You could see that she was churning numbers in her head, trying to calculate what was not there.

"Well, I've never been fired or involved in a car accident during those times. But, I was close, at least with regard to the car accident," she replied.

I quickly delved into the issue at hand, knowing that this was the crux of the problem, her continual catastrophizing.

I started: "When we do the calculations, the odds of either of those happening are nil. You mentioned that there was an 80% probability of your termination and car crash when the actual, 'real-life' calculations show that this has never occurred. So even though you worried that your fears would come true sometime during those 600 sleepless nights, they never actually did. Do you see that?"

Ava remained silent, but you could see her smirk.

"When you put it that way, I guess the entire thing seems a bit silly. But in my mind, it's an ever-present danger, as if these things are certainly bound to occur. In fact, I can see it so clearly and imagine those scenes repetitively in my mind. It's so exhausting. I feel like I'm living a double life, one in this world and one in this other world, where I imagine things happening. I don't make sense, do I?" she apologetically questioned.

"You certainly make sense. Actually, it's very logical and shows that you're a real thinker and problem solver, but unfortunately, that doesn't work well for a restful sleep," I replied. "As humans, fortunately or unfortunately, we are able to think and project things into the future. And therein lies the problem, because we envision things and create all sorts of prophesies that never come to light. And, even the best of us are probably a tinge more pessimistic than optimistic, hence the need to make things appear worse than they actually are."

"Yes, I certainly fit that definition. I've never been able to think about the positive, only the negative. I guess that's why I'm so depressed," she said.

"Well, the topic of depression is multifaceted and too difficult to disentangle now. But there is probably a chemical imbalance that, with your changed circumstances, brought on your depression. Taking an antidepressant is a good idea for you. That will at least improve your depression. But your sleep is just as important," I said.

"I can see that very clearly now," she replied, a little more energetically than she had previously.

"I have a little exercise for you to do when you can't sleep at night," I said.

"What's that?" she quizzically asked.

"Whenever you can't fall asleep, I want you to counter your catastrophic thoughts of 'If I don't fall asleep, I will crash my car or lose my job' with 'That is very unlikely with all the stats that the sleep doctor presented to me. In fact, the chances are nil or close to nil.'"

"That's great to know. I think that will help me a lot. I often think of those things when I'm lying in bed for hours," she said.

"Well, that's only the beginning. I think we may have to work on your sleep hygiene, as well as on concepts of stimulus control and sleep restriction. We have many more weeks of cognitive behavioral therapy ahead of us, but the concept of catastrophizing is an important one that saves a lot of people from the perils of their insomnia."

"I see. Yes, I'm on board for this cognitive therapy. I don't want to take any sleeping medications if I don't have to," she quickly retorted. "My previous psychiatrist was giving me a concoction of drugs. I felt like she was giving me the key to her drugstore. If I weren't so dismayed about my insomnia, it would actually have been quite funny. I really appreciate this drug-free approach to my problem."

"Well, that's what I'm here for," I excitedly replied. "So, two more concepts before we finish this session. These concepts may be counterintuitive and directly opposed to the one I just told you about, but test it out and see what you think."

I told her about the performance anxiety that often accompanies those with insomnia, whose entire thought is related to falling asleep and not "performing" this task. I went on to suggest that performance anxiety not only relates to daily tasks but also to sleep. Sleep is a natural process and cannot be dictated. You cannot tell someone to fall asleep at a moment's notice—on demand—because a certain chemical—adenosine—has to build to a certain extent before one falls asleep. I told her to think of adenosine as a natural anesthetic that accumulates the longer one doesn't sleep. Eventually, sleep will come naturally when someone hasn't slept for a while. It's inevitable. But performance anxiety complicates things because it runs opposite to this buildup.

"So, what should I do when this happens, when I have such an anxiety?" she replied.

"Well, don't forget about the concept of catastrophizing that we just discussed in length. But you can also add in a different mantra to trick your brain in a way. If, when you start worrying, you introduce the mantra of 'to hell with it all' or 'fuck it all,' you can find peace in your worries. Essentially, if you're already thinking that your life is gone or will go wrong, you have nothing left to lose. This approach pushes the catastrophization to such an extreme degree that, when it comes time to worry, you've already encountered the worst case scenario in your mind and come to terms with it. It's easy to fall into a cycle of worrying, and admittedly, this new concept will take a bit more time to sharpen, but it's a good tool for your arsenal, nonetheless."

In my years of conducting cognitive behavioral sessions, I have found this concept to be more difficult to grasp but I think that it is one that is helpful, as some will respond to it better than catastrophizing. Most people have difficulty imagining their lives as "messed-up" because that is what they are trying so desperately to avoid. But when you have already made this a foregone conclusion, you have already let go, so why not use it to your advantage and reverse it? Letting go is an important aspect of insomnia in that sleep cannot be forced. It needs to occur naturally and seamlessly, like the adenosine that accumulates and lets you naturally fall asleep.

"I may have to think about this concept for a while," Ava quietly said, "but I sort of get it. It's like my life has already gone wrong, or will, so what's the point of worrying about it?"

"Precisely. There is another concept that's related to this, which, again, is very counterintuitive."

"And what is that called?"

You could tell that she was getting frustrated at this point, with so many strategies thrust upon her.

"Well, it's reverse psychology, really. As I told you, performance is a big problem for those who feel they cannot sleep in a timely manner. The lights are out and everyone else is sleeping, and, like an indirect cue, they are told that they should be sleeping, too."

"Exactly. I usually feel like that. Like I've been given a task in the office and can't perform it."

"Yes! So, the same goes with sleep. You cannot tell yourself to fall asleep. However, what you can do is to tell yourself to not fall asleep."

"What did you just say? That I should tell myself *not* to fall asleep."

"Exactly. That's the power of the technique called paradoxical intention. It doesn't work for everyone, and it may not work for you, but it's another powerful strategy. Studies have shown that patients who use this strategy fall asleep faster with less anxiety."

"Can I mix these strategies or focus on one?"

"Good question. Initially, I would focus on cognitive therapy, because it has been studied the longest and it's the most robust, but if you feel that after a while this doesn't work for you, feel free to give the other techniques a shot. Everyone's sleep is not created equally, so see what works for you."

"Great. I like the idea of paradoxical intention, because half the time, I'm telling myself to fall asleep and am under extreme anxiety to make this occur, kind of like passing a law school exam. Contrary to what others think, I don't do well under pressure. Sleep has become another exam that I have to pass, and it has become so tiring."

"Precisely. Let's finish on that note, because I think we've covered a lot of ground today," I replied.

She averted her gaze before confronting me directly. You could tell that she agreed about ending this session.

"This has been very helpful. Thank you, doctor. I feel more confident now. Those concepts really resonate with me."

"We'll continue with this cognitive restructuring in our next session, but I'm glad that we got the basics down. I'll see you next time, and, hopefully, your sleep will have improved by then," I said.

Ava thanked me again and, as she left my office, she turned into the wrong hallway. I could see that she was still thinking about these concepts, and her distraction actually reassured me.

☾

Sleep Pearls

Ava's narrative showed how catastrophization is an immense barrier to good sleep. It enlarges the problem at hand, in this case insomnia, so that everything that flows from it is magnified unrealistically. Ava made herself believe that if she did not obtain good sleep, she'd get fired from her job as an attorney or be involved in a car accident, both of which never occurred. The key here was to show her that such thinking was skewed because the probability that those things would happen were nil, given her past record. We had to cognitively restructure her negative thinking patterns, so she would understand that they were unrealistic.

Another tool we used here was combatting performance anxiety using paradoxical intention; Ava had immense anxiety about "performing well" when going to sleep. For her, it had become another exam to conquer, just like in law school. As we learned, you cannot force yourself to go to sleep. However, forcing yourself to stay awake may actually work in this instance, because there is no anxiety in doing that. Furthermore, with paradoxical intention, you're confronting your fear of not being able to sleep head-on, so it no longer exerts power over you. You're essentially breaking that fear cycle and powerfully combating insomnia on your own terms.

Ava returned to the clinic a month later, more cheerful and relaxed. She had restructured her thought patterns so that her dilemmas weren't life-and-death or success-and-failure propositions. In short, she did not catastrophize the things that could happen if she didn't sleep well. Ava realized that her previous thoughts were unrealistic. Moreover, she was successfully taking an antidepressant and tackling her depression, which had negatively added to that catastrophization.

Case 3

Stephen

Traumatic Memories and Nightmares

H E WASN'T REALLY THERE, HE EVENTUALLY TOLD ME
after I had first met Stephen in consultation. Or, rather, he was
there, at the right time, at the right place, but everything was horrific.
Like really, really horrific. He never experienced the event because, at
the moment that he saw them—the fallen—he was already outside of
himself, looking in, as it were, to see himself as the business consultant
who had shown up late to a meeting in which he was speaking and
missed a tragic death—his own.

Stephen explained it this way: "I was supposed to present a talk to a
group of businessmen, ironically, on the topic of speculation and gam-
bling, on how even a small change in an equation could dramatically
change the results and reap unimaginable benefits."

His message for this aging company was to take a chance and implement a change that would harness the power of the internet and affect
the millions who were using it. In other words, he would tell them, this
opportunity would only happen now, if they acted shrewdly and set
the ball in motion. It was now or never. They had to be at the right place
at the right time, and the time was now. Yes, they had to be lucky and
speculative, but they had to look at the data and understand that this
change would fundamentally and assuredly prove to be a positive one.

He was rehearsing this phrase, and the variation of this idea, over and over. It had to be just right and delivered just so. This was a chance to wow one of the biggest companies in New York. It was his big opportunity to embark successfully on his fledgling career as a business consultant.

So, on the morning of September 11, 2001, Stephen energetically awoke from his firm bed, with luxurious 500-thread count linens, and was excited to deliver his mantra to this group of successful committee members. He had splayed his business suit, shirt, and tie on the ottoman in his hotel room at the Marriott Hotel, which was positioned between the Twin Towers. He knew that he would be excited on the morning of his talk, so he had judiciously prepared his attire for that day. He was always a great sleeper, he said, but hadn't slept that well on that particular night due to his excitement. Regardless, he was always energized when he woke up from sleep. "You couldn't find a better sleeper than me. I fell asleep at the drop of a pin and couldn't be roused, even with a loud bang. But everything changed after 9/11."

Stephen went back to the day of the attack. He had tried on his dress shirt and suit. He thought that he looked very professional and handsome. He had brought two ties with him from Ohio, one a basic blue and the other patterned with a blue, bold paisley print. He had deliberated over these two ties obsessively. Everything had to be perfect for his big chance. He had initially tried on the plain blue tie and, after reaching the lobby of the hotel, decided that it was all wrong. Wasn't his message supposed to be that change is good, that unconventional techniques yield the biggest results? Why was he wearing a basic blue tie, one that signaled conventionality and the mundane? Yes, his suit and tie projected professionalism, but he needed his tie to signal that he wasn't afraid to be a bit different. He took the elevator to his room on the 11th floor, Room 1111, and speedily changed to the other tie. Despite his swiftness, he would be arriving at the very start of the meeting, although he had anticipated arriving at least 15 minutes in advance to prepare himself and calm his nerves.

He took the elevator down to the lobby, exited it, and sensed a sudden movement in the building. Was this an earthquake, here in New York City? This didn't seem possible, he thought. He exited the building with a few others, and that's when he saw it. The sudden burst of flashing lights, the debris, people falling, resembling miniscule cartoon figures. None of this seemed real, he thought. He was looking at the horror before him but couldn't register any of it. Images flickered here and there, but he felt that he was experiencing this outside himself. Although he didn't want to look, he was fixated on the scene. He could hear shouts, cries, fire trucks, and police sirens. He had never experienced such a sensory overload, as if he had been blasted with a gun of images directed at him alone. He even felt something on his face, but just let it work its way to his mouth. He licked it. It tasted like dirt. He was okay with that. At least, it wasn't blood. The police made their way to the crowd that had now increased in size. They directed the bystanders to make their way away from the Towers, away from the hotel. He remembered being told to "Get the hell away from here. Just keep moving steadily and calmly but go and get away! Now."

It's 2007 now, but Stephen thinks obsessively about how he survived the disaster when he should have clearly been in that building, being blown to smithereens or falling to his death amid a blazing explosion. How could this seemingly arbitrary decision of changing a tie have led him from death to salvation? He said that he felt guilty for being one of the few who escaped from their fates that day. He *should've* been at that meeting with the board members, he *should've* died, but he didn't. Although he should have felt grateful for his survival, all he could feel was guilt while seeing the bodies falling incessantly before him. He had heard of other people who had missed their deaths, like chef Michael Lomonaco of Windows on the World who had decided to purchase new glasses in the shopping plaza under the World Trade Center. His 72 coworkers were killed, but Lomonaco had fatefully survived. Stephen thought that the entire thing was unfair. Was this chance or was there a plan for him by a higher power? He wasn't actually religious, but this experience had made him rethink his beliefs.

What made this experience so unreal for him were the unrelenting images of the fallen victims, those plunging hundreds of feet to their deaths. Those were the images that wouldn't go away, and hadn't gone away for the past 6 years. He hadn't slept peacefully since that fateful day. A year after the attack, he ultimately decided to quit his job as a business consultant, leave the industrial landscape of Cleveland, Ohio, and pursue his passion of being an actor. He couldn't let this chance of fulfilling his dream get away from him once more.

At the present, he was just making ends meet, working as a waiter in a restaurant in downtown Los Angeles, while going to auditions that hadn't landed him anywhere. He said that he never really liked his profession as a consultant anyway, and, now that he had escaped death, he should pursue what he always enjoyed—acting. He had been given a second chance at life, and he would take advantage of this opportunity. But despite being happy in this way, his sleep was never the same. Where once he was the envy of others regarding his sleep, he now cursed those who slept well. At dinner parties he had recently attended, he couldn't even hear anything related to sleep. It always conjured the memories of his perfect sleep, the one he knew he could never attain again.

Stephen said he had been consulting with a clinical psychologist here in Los Angeles and undergoing eye movement desensitization and reprocessing (EMDR) therapy. This is a type of therapy in which the person being treated is asked to recall traumatic images while the therapist directs the patient to undergo repeated eye movements. The theory underlying this is that the patient's underlying negative thoughts and behaviors are the result of unprocessed memories that need to come to the forefront in order for the patient to process them and confront their demons, so to speak. In the case of post-traumatic stress disorder (PTSD), information processing has been halted in the memory networks, so the goal of EMDR is to access and reprocess these memories. Stephen had also been prescribed prazosin, a medication for hypertension and urinary retention that is used to treat nightmares and PTSD symptoms. But it hadn't really alleviated his suffering. This medication had helped many veterans with the symptoms of their PTSD, but it had only tempered Stephen's. He felt that no one had adequately dealt with his sleep issues, when the images of fallen victims would overwhelm his senses. He could smell the debris from the fire, he could feel the warmth of that burning, and it would all come rushing back to him.

This was a lot to deal with. I could sense that this 28-year-old ex-business consultant, who was now a fledgling actor, had once been carefree, but he was now shackled by these sensations that would force themselves upon him at the most inopportune time, namely when he wanted to sleep. He was afraid to sleep because the images of the fallen would appear on at least a weekly basis. He "feared" sleep, as he acknowledged to me. Sleep enervated him. He felt more tired when he slept. He was tired of being tired.

We decided to start on a nonpharmacological treatment for him called image rehearsal therapy (IRT), a behavioral intervention that involves rewriting the "script" of one's nightmares and rehearsing this modified and less problematic version. It's not considered a component of cognitive behavioral therapy for insomnia, per se, but it is directed therapy for those who are undergoing nightmares. The nightmare sufferers are encouraged to rewrite their dreams in whatever way they'd like (i.e. changing the ending, rewriting the beginning, showing themselves to be active participants in thwarting it) and rehearsing this new dream. I instructed Stephen to rewrite the script in a way compatible with his beliefs and comfort level. The dream did not necessarily need to be positive or triumphant but rather a dream that worked for him in any way he saw fit. The important thing was that he should take an active role in reformulating this dream. This behavioral strategy of rescripting one's nightmares has proven to be effective in the long run while allowing the sufferer to also confront the nightmare or post-traumatic issue during their waking life. The goal of IRT is to provide control over whatever disturbing images or senses the sufferers encounter during their nightmares or post-traumatic thoughts. By re-scripting certain scenes in their nightmares, they are able to exert a control that they never had while the event was unfolding; they now can do something about a situation over which they had once been powerless.

After a few sessions together, Stephen had rescripted his nightmare quite nicely, but not in the way I had expected. He had become a true hero in the situation by warning everyone in the Twin Towers about the impending attack. How had he done this? He had written the script to make himself the double agent, the asset, who knew about the attack from the terrorist attackers themselves. He had gathered intel that the bombing would occur and had conveyed this information to the US government. The details of how this had occurred were less relevant than what he hoped to do with the information. So, on that fateful day, although the Twin Towers had been dismantled, no one had actually been in the buildings. However, Stephen himself had not changed his routine. He was staying at the hotel and had played the part of wanting to present his strategy to the board (which he knew he would not do). He had walked outside of the hotel, though, and had felt the debris and smell of the smoke. But, when he looked up, he saw no one crying for help, no one jumping from the building, no clothes being used as parachutes. In the end, he had thwarted Al-Qaeda's plans and been the hero. He told me that he had scripted this nightmare this way because he couldn't dismiss the fact that 9/11 had happened. It had, and he couldn't just erase this important history, which had left an indelible mark on so many individuals and families. To dismiss this important history was sacrilegious. Instead, he had to rescript this so that no one would be hurt or killed inside the building. Sure, there would still be deaths from the crash itself and the victims on the planes, but he had to make the dream as realistic as possible while saving as many people as he could. In this way, Stephen had become a true hero, and his (active) actions had transformed his once passive role. Over the course of 3 months (because meaningful improvements occur over time), Stephen had memorized this script so well that he had become an impressive actor in his dreams. Fortuitously, he had even managed to land a few small television roles for which he had recently auditioned. He was sure that rescripting his nightmare and becoming an active hero had provided him with the confidence to become that hero everyone wanted to emulate.

Subsequently, Stephen and I delved into the matter further to address his post-traumatic issues in a larger framework. We implemented exposure, rescripting, and relaxation therapy (ERRT), which is a multicomponent protocol for nightmares and PTSD. ERRT involves immersion in education about sleep and nightmares, sleep hygiene, exposure to nightmares, nightmare rescripting (as we had previously discussed), and relaxation techniques. In other words, we brought all aspects of his trauma together, along with the IRT with which he had seen much success.

During our last consultation, I could see that Stephen was transformed. He was no longer that timid individual who was unsure of himself and his capabilities. He had landed a few good roles and was working as a waiter. Most importantly, he was now sleeping about 6 to 7 hours per night and no longer had a fear of falling asleep. Although he acknowledged that this therapy had taken about 6 months to complete, he no longer had the nightmares that had initially brought him in. If anything, he felt like he could tackle any personal issues in his waking life, too. The techniques he had learned from IRT and ERRT had provided him with the impetus to "crush" anything that stood in his way, including his auditions. He was happy, and he was smiling.

(

Sleep Pearls

As Stephen's case reveals, image rehearsal therapy (IRT) is an excellent way to deal with trauma, PTSD, and nightmares without the use of medications. As the term implies, one is actually rehearsing the trauma or nightmare that is fueling the distressed sleep and providing it with a comfortable resolution. More importantly, IRT provides the type of control that was missing in the first place and substitutes the passive object for the active subject. IRT can take some time to master, but with patience and practice, it can be an invaluable tool for tackling these kinds of scenarios.

Savannah

Delayed Sleep Phase Syndrome
and Circadian Rhythms

HER NAME WAS SAVANNAH, LIKE THE CITY IN GEORGIA. She was a bright 23-year-old woman. Just 1 year after graduating university, she had landed a fairly respectable position as an assistant writer for a web drama series set in the 1980s. She didn't resemble a southerner in style or voice. Far from it. Her hair was tousled and wavy. She wore a slashed neck graffiti T-shirt, with the logo of the band *The Strokes* emblazoned on it. She spoke like a Valley girl from the 1980s, although her speech and accent weren't quite feigned. She had blonde hair that was pieced together in various vibrant colors, some pink, some blue, some green. If one didn't know better, they would think she was showing up to an audition for a Cyndi Lauper music video—it was that glaring and imitative.

She was a couple of hours late to her appointment, which was originally scheduled for 11 a.m. Although my assistant had told her the office had a 30-minute window before appointments were cancelled so as to give the other patients ample time for their own appointments, she insisted that she be seen.

"You don't understand how important this appointment is to me," I could hear her tell my assistant. "I've been waiting 2 months for this and I simply need to see the doctor. My life is in shambles and it's falling apart slowly every day. *Please.* I'll even wait after hours if I have to. I haven't been held in traffic or anything. The reason I'm late is my sleep disorder," she continued.

My assistant had come to my office to explain the situation and I instantly recognized the diagnosis I would be confronting. Missing late morning or early afternoon appointments, without a clear reason, was one of its hallmarks. I told my assistant I'd see Savannah. This was no fault of her own. Her circadian rhythms were out of sync, something she had no control over.

Once her vitals were taken, I walked into the exam room. She was frantically texting someone, so occupied with her iPhone that she didn't realize that I had entered the room.

I opened the door to the exam room, greeted her, and initiated our conversation.

"Hi, Ms. LeBlanc."

"Oh. Hi, doctor. Please call me Savannah."

She was surprised, as if I'd walked into the room while she was doing something furtively.

"I'm just about to finish this text. So sorry. It looks like I'll be late to a couple more appointments today. I just have to let the others know."

"That's fine. Let's get started, though."

"Yes. I'm so, so sorry for being late. You don't understand. I'm late *all* the time, through no fault of my own. It's like my body is this robot and I have no control over when it wants to wake up. *Please* help me."

She emphasized some of her words while drawing the rest out, as if to show that she really was in need of some assistance. One could hear the desperation in her voice, loud and clear.

"What can I do for you, Savannah? Although I can guess why you're here."

"You can?"

"Let's just say that I've seen my fair share of this disorder throughout my years of practicing sleep medicine. You're not alone."

Her smile widened, like she'd just been handed a present she wasn't expecting.

"You have? You can really diagnose me just like that? Please, do tell."

"Okay. If I'm on the right track, you've had this sleep problem since you were an adolescent and you've never been able to sleep on time, when you were told to, right?"

"Yes, that's exactly right. My sleep problems started in high school when I was expected to go to sleep at a certain time and wake up for my classes, which were too early for me. Way too early. During that time, I went to bed at 9 p.m. and wasn't able to fall asleep until midnight, sometimes later. It was insane, absolutely insane. I had to be up by 6 a.m. to get ready for school, but most days, I just couldn't wake up. Swear to god, I really couldn't. My parents attributed this problem to my casual attitude and my laziness, but I seriously *could not* wake up. It was as if my body were a magnet glued to the bed. It was so surreal. They would call my name: *Savannah! Savannah!* and, for the life of me, I couldn't move. That's the best I can describe it. Of course, my grades suffered in the process, but I aced my SATs and landed at Brown to study semiotics and film theory. My parents were never satisfied with me during high school, though. They begged me to go and see a sleep doctor then, but I resisted that. I thought that it was just me, and that I was the problem. I didn't think anything could be done about it. When you've had this problem ever since you can remember, it just totally becomes part of you. Does that make sense?"

"It does. Did your sleep improve at the university? Were you able to attend your classes on time? Did you feel happier?"

"Ah. That's the funny thing. I did pretty well in my classes at university, but that's because I was able to select my classes. I felt better, and my mood drastically changed. It was as if I were given this new life that I had always imagined but could never attain. I selected my courses mainly in the afternoon, so that was cool. However, I had a few morning classes that I was required to take because those were only offered in the morning and I couldn't attend those. Totally couldn't. In fact, for one of my history classes, I never even saw the inside of that classroom. No joke. I bought the notes for the class and listened to the audio lectures. Thankfully, it was a large class and the professor didn't call roll. So, I somehow scraped by. But it was quite a feat. It was like reliving my nightmarish high school days all over again. And it was no fun."

"I see. Well, let me ask you this. Why are you seeing a sleep physician after all these years? Have your circumstances changed?"

"Well, yeah, that's the thing. During my senior year in university, I was offered this great gig to be one of the writers of this web series set in the '80s, and it was like a dream. But, when I realized the writers met in the morning, like around 10 a.m., my dreams shattered a bit. How would I be able to get up that early, which, I realize for most is a 'normal' time? There was no way I could do that, given my precedent."

She used her hands for air quotes, and then continued.

"I told myself that I could muster the strength to get up early because this was my dream, after all. My mind would take over and my adrenaline would surge. Well, it worked for about a week, but I was a total wreck. I could tell that the other writers were noticing this, so I opted to finally see a doctor. This is my third week on the job and I'm absolutely terrified that I'll totally mess this up . . . So, doctor, what do I have? It is something that can be treated?"

"Yes, absolutely. You have a classic case of delayed sleep phase syndrome, a circadian disorder, where your timeline is out of sync with the majority of people's. Only about 10% of the population has this sleep disorder, so I guess you're one of the select few."

"Lucky me!"

She made a facetious grin and continued to listen. I went on with my sleeping lesson.

"Believe it or not, this disorder serves some people very well. These 'night owls,' as we like to call them, are most creative at night, so this circadian misalignment actually serves a purpose for them. And, because there doesn't appear to be a problem when these night owls have adapted well to their sleep disorder, everyone is happy. Like when you went to college and were able to adapt to your class schedule by purposefully selecting courses that agreed with your rhythm."

"Yeah, totally!"

Savannah became animated and listened more attentively, as if she was learning how to construct this jigsaw puzzle that had eluded her for such a long time.

"The problem arises when the schedules of most people don't align with yours, which is, unfortunately, the majority. If you could live in a world of night owls, you'd succeed very well. But because we're in the land of the normal animals, you struggle."

"I know it. It totally SUCKS. So, what's the solution?"

"It's actually not so difficult, but you have to adhere to a pretty strict regimen."

"Yeah, I'll do whatever. I really want to keep this gig. If I mess up now, no one will hire me."

"Let's not get ahead of ourselves. You're also catastrophizing your problem, which we'll discuss in another session. That is a tendency to inflate things and make them life-or-death propositions. But, for now, I think our first step is realigning your circadian rhythms. To do this, I will need to know your sleep habits, like when you actually sleep, if given the opportunity to sleep at whatever time you'd like. And, also, what time you'd naturally awake if no one pestered you. Basically, I want you to tell me your 'dream' sleep schedule."

"Well, that's easy. If only I could sleep like I used to in college, that'd be heaven!"

"I'll get you there."

"That'd be so wonderful. I would love to sleep at 2 a.m. and wake up at 10 or 11 a.m. I mean, before, in high school, I would get into bed at 9 p.m. and not go to sleep until midnight. And then I had to wake up at 6 a.m. to shower and eat breakfast before I left for school. As I said before, that was an absolute nightmare. Most of the time, I had no time for breakfast, and, as a result, I felt super hungry and about to pass out in class. That feeling of being dazed and hungry also affected my grades and participation in class. Everyone threw the word *insomnia* at me, but I intuitively knew in my guts that it was not the correct diagnosis."

"Yup. It's not insomnia because, with insomnia, it doesn't matter what time you sleep. You would still feel restless even if you went to bed at 2 a.m. The problem that you have is different. You can actually sleep if you go to bed at the time that aligns with your circadian rhythm."

"Exactly! That I can do. I have no problem sleeping if I go to bed at my desired sleep time."

"Okay. So, now, my lesson becomes a bit mathematical."

"What do you mean? I was never good at math. I majored in film theory and semiotics at Brown, after all."

I laughed, realizing that I shouldn't have introduced math into our conversation so quickly. As I've gathered through the years, most insomniacs don't like the concept of math when discussing their sleep problems. That's just an observation, not a fact.

"It's not math, per se, but some simple calculations."

"Oh, I can definitely do that."

"Before we embark on these calculations, let me explain some other concepts to you. The first is dim light melatonin. Our brain starts secreting melatonin in response to darkness, as our body and mind are ready to go to sleep. It's called the hormone of darkness. Darkness promotes secretion of this hormone while light inhibits it, which is also important that you taper use of your phone and other electronic equipment that emits blue light, especially once you're winding down to go to sleep. Blue light suppresses the body's release of melatonin. While this may be helpful during the day, it becomes a problem at night when we're trying to sleep. That means no more texts and use of your iPhone for a couple of hours before you go to bed. Light is not good for your sleep. Actually, light is not good for anyone's sleep, but in particular, those with circadian disorders demonstrate greater sensitivity of the circadian system to the phase-delaying effects of light. In other words, your sleep is more influenced by light than it would be for those who don't have a delayed sleep phase."

"Oh, I see. But that's going to be difficult, given what I do. I'm always getting texts by the group of writers that I work with about ideas they have regarding the script we're working with during that week."

"I think your sleep is more important, so just let them know that you're trying to improve your sleep and your doctor told you to stop the use of electronics after a certain time. If you'd like, I can give you a note explaining that. People usually take it very seriously if you hand them a doctor's note."

"Yeah, for sure. That could work. Otherwise, they'll think I'm trying to ignore them and slack off, especially since I just started this job."

"Well, we don't want that."

"Okay, what else do I need to do?"

"Like I said, we need to do a bit of a calculation to figure out your need to get sunlight and melatonin, two very important *zeitgebers* for realigning your circadian rhythm. *Zeitgeber* is a German term that means 'time giver' and refers to the environmental variables that act as circadian time cues. The light and dark cycle is the most important zeitgeber, but other stimuli, such as melatonin, also function this way."

"That's kind of interesting. So how do we use this information to fix my sleep? I don't need theory—I had enough of that in college. I need something practical."

"So, you told me that, if left to your own devices, you would go to bed at 2 a.m. and wake up at 10 or 11 a.m. Is that correct?

"Yes, unfortunately."

"We need to do some math here. Your dim light melatonin onset, then, or your DLMO as we sleep doctors call it, is 2 hours before your 'natural' sleep time. The DLMO is defined as the start of the melatonin production in the evening during dim light conditions. As the name suggests, it is the onset of melatonin production and release. We use this to determine when you should take melatonin."

"I'm a little confused. I've been taking melatonin about 30 minutes prior to sleep. Is that not correct? I thought that's when you need to take it."

"That's correct if you have classic insomnia. However, you have delayed sleep phase syndrome, and that requires that melatonin be taken much earlier, about 5 hours prior to your DLMO, because that timing, based on numerous research studies, will provide you with the best advancement of your circadian clock. Based on your natural sleep time, your DLMO is about midnight. So, you should be taking mela-tonin 5 hours before that, at 7 p.m."

"Whoa, really? That's insane. I've never heard that before. So early? Are you sure?"

"Yup. Call it what you will, but that is one of the ways we can advance your sleep, so that you can sleep earlier. A 3-mg dose will usually suf-fice. Taking any more than that will not help, and it can make you groggy. Some have suggested that a 0.5 mg dose also works, although in my experience, a 3-mg dose is optimal."

"I can do that. I've been taking a 10-mg dose in the supermarket and, you're right, it's giving me some very vivid dreams and I'm very groggy in the morning. At times, I feel this out-of-body experience, especially if I'm very sleep-deprived."

"You may also consider purchasing ultra-pure melatonin, which offers continuous release and absorption. Basically, this form replicates the way in which the body releases and absorbs melatonin."

"I'll definitely do that."

"However, the most effective and potent *zeitgeber* that we have at our disposal is natural light, which we can greatly use to our advantage."

"How do we do that?

"So, just as we calculated your DLMO to determine the time you should take melatonin, we can do the same thing with the timing of your exposure to light."

"Please continue."

"You say that you naturally wake up at 10 or 11 a.m. So let's take the more conservative time and say that your ideal wake-up time is 11 a.m. Our core body temperature starts to drop 2 hours before we go to sleep, coinciding with the release of melatonin. It reaches its lowest level 2 hours before your natural wake-up time now, which, for you, is 9 a.m."

"Okay. So why is 9 a.m. so important?"

"It's important because at that time, or shortly thereafter, I want you to get natural sunlight, or if the weather is cloudy, to use a light-box for at least 30 minutes. At that hour, the light will advance your sleep and move it to an earlier time, so that you can awaken at an earlier time. We'll continue to do this weekly until we arrive at a schedule that works with your work schedule."

"Really? That seems almost magical, as if the sun is a sorceress."

"It's not that dramatic. The key piece to remember is that a portion of your brain called the hypothalamus is the central pacemaker of your circadian system. It's your natural alarm clock. When light conveys itself through your eyes, through the retina, it transmits a message to your hypothalamus that morning has arrived and it's time to reset your circadian rhythm. In a sense, you're fooling the brain to get the outcome you want."

"I like this idea a lot, it feels like I'm outwitting my circadian rhythm."

"I'm glad you think so—all the more power to you."

"So, what do I do after that?"

"Well, take the melatonin at the time that we talked about at 7 p.m., do your thing, sleep as best as you can, set your alarm at 9 a.m., get up, and get natural sunlight for at least 30 minutes. The exposure duration should be anywhere from 30 to 90 minutes, but you may be time-constrained and only get light for 30 minutes. You have to be at the writers' meeting at 10 a.m., if I recall correctly?"

"Yeah, that's right, so it's cutting it close."

"Take a quick shower after your walk outside and head to work. It's not going to be that easy at first, but the goal is to advance your sleep onset and wake-up time by 30 minutes each week, until you reach your goal of 8 a.m. As I said, it won't be painless, but you will eventually wake up and feel rested at the hour that you'd like."

"Well, what if I get up earlier this week, let's say at 8 a.m., and try to get sunlight? Won't that be a faster way to "advance" my circadian rhythm? I'll do whatever it takes, even if it means waking up that early."

Savannah's eyes were lit up, as if she had discovered a secret. She wanted results quickly. Now! I looked at her fiery eyes and continued, trying to temper her newfound wisdom just slightly.

"That's a great point, Savannah. However, if you obtain sunlight earlier than the 2 hours before your natural wake-up time, you can actually delay your circadian rhythm. The sunlight has to arrive precisely at or just slightly after 9 a.m. Conversely, if you get sunlight at 10 a.m., your circadian rhythm will only advance negligibly. So, it's very important that you adhere to this precise regimen."

"I see."

Savannah's hope had somewhat dissipated, but she was still excited about the prospect for improvement.

"Let me ask you this, doctor. When it gets light outside, do I wear my sunglasses? It tends to get very bright here in Los Angeles at that time of day."

"Great point, and one I may not have mentioned. No, you must not wear sunglasses. The entire point is to get the light into the retinae. Wearing sunglasses will not accomplish this."

"Got it. You were also talking about a light box. Can you tell me more about this? It sounds like such a cool gadget."

"It *is* a cool gadget. The light box simulates light. It's basically fake light—not as good as the real thing—but it works, especially if you're in a location where you can't get light like we get here almost year-round, like in Seattle or Stockholm. The box should be full-spectrum at 10,000 lux, and it should be situated about 2 feet from you. It's very important to remember, you cannot look at it directly. You can place it adjacent to your computer, for instance, so the light hits your eyes indirectly. But you should be aware of some side effects. Initially, you may experience eye strain, headache, and nausea. If you have a history of mania, which your questionnaire indicates that you don't, the use of the light box is not recommended because it can actually precipitate a manic episode. Also, if you have any disease of the retinae or cataracts, which, again, you don't have, the use of a light box is not recommended. In short, always try to get natural sunlight and use the box only for those circumstances when you cannot."

"Got it!"

"Fantastic. Now let's put these tools to use and have you return in a couple of weeks. I would also like you to keep a sleep journal to accurately depict the times you get up, obtain sunlight, take melatonin, and so forth—basically the strategies that we already discussed. This will help determine when you should get light and take melatonin, especially because we'll be changing these times slowly every week."

"Oh, right. That makes perfect sense. The sooner I do this, the sooner I can get my career going. I really want this to work out! Thank you for your help. I really needed this."

"No problem. I'll see you here in a couple of weeks. We can discuss your progress then. I'm confident that you'll be sleeping and feeling much better soon if you take these steps."

She donned her bright fluorescent green sunglasses and headed out the door. Before doing so, she turned around and gave a smile, as if she was sure of herself, her multicolored hair swinging with that movement.

She exclaimed, "I can wear my sunglasses now, because it's not morning."

Her dream of being a successful scriptwriter was palpable and within reach.

I don't know what I was expecting when Savannah returned several weeks later to my office. In my experience, I've found that patients are either frustrated by the regimen that has been thrust upon them or they are pleasantly surprised that sleep science was able to guide them to their ideal sleep schedule. Fortunately, for me and Savannah, the latter turned out to be the outcome.

I heard Savannah strut into the office with her high-heeled boots while I was walking down the corridor to my office. She was exhilarated and full of energy. Her appointment time was 10 a.m., and she was actually early. She was donned again in her '80s attire, this time with a ripped T-shirt for The Go-Gos' *Beauty and the Beat*. She had dyed her tousled motley-colored hair blonde. She was smiling.

"Hello, Savannah. How are you?"

"As you can tell, I'm actually doing really, really well. I can't believe that I was living with this circadian problem all my life without realizing it. If I had known this earlier, my time in high school would've been so, so different, not to mention the interactions I had with my parents about my sleep."

"Well, we've tackled the problem now. I wouldn't ponder on everything that could've happened if we had tackled the issue then. It doesn't serve you well. Think about the future and change that. Dwelling in the past never helped anyone.

"Yeah, I guess you're right. I'll be a futurist."

"So, please tell me about what helped and what didn't."

"Well, the first week was tough. Getting up at 9 a.m. was not easy, but I had a solution and a goal that I needed to conquer. I don't think I could've done this if I didn't have a deadline and my dream job both looming over me."

She flashed a large grin and continued.

"Like I said, the first 3 days were tough, but I went outside and got about 30 minutes of sunlight, without sunglasses, of course, and headed to work. I was groggy at work but had told the script supervisor about my 'intervention,' so she understood."

"Good. How about the melatonin?"

"Oh, yes. I'm now taking that at 7 p.m. instead of 30 minutes prior to sleep, as I used to do. I'm also taking a smaller dose and, pleasantly enough, don't feel the grogginess of the larger dose."

"Great. It appears that you're progressing as you should. Now, I have to caution you that delayed sleep phase syndrome has a high rate of relapse and you must keep to your regimen. The night owl in you is so ingrained that if you falter a bit, it could rear its head. Unless, of course, you want that or have a job that requires that nocturnal activity."

"I figured that. No, at this point, I'm fully committed to making this work. I think I can maintain this schedule."

"Fantastic. Well, I'm very proud of your perseverance, Savannah. I recognize that none of this has been easy for you."

"Thank you again. I really appreciate all that you've done for me."

She genuinely smiled, and I could tell that she was really pleased with what she had accomplished in such a short time.

Sleep Pearls

It is important to distinguish delayed sleep phase syndrome (DSPS) from insomnia because the treatment for each is so very different. Often, when an individual cannot sleep, it is assumed that they have insomnia, as in Savannah's case. However, the critical question to ask yourself is whether you can fall asleep or maintain sleep easily if you go to bed later. If the answer is yes, you most likely don't suffer from insomnia but rather from one of its imitators, such as DSPS. As you've come to realize, DSPS stems from a circadian misalignment, so treatment for this disorder is different from that for insomnia. Now, you may have a combination of insomnia and DSPS if you retire to bed later but still cannot fall asleep. Treatment for this condition needs to be directed first to DSPS and then to insomnia through the CBT-I program outlined in the second part of this book.

Case 5

Allen and Izzie

Obstructive Sleep Apnea and Environmental Sleep Disorder

ZZIE AND HER HUSBAND, ALLEN, CAME TO SEE ME IN my sleep clinic. As healthy, trendy, and well-groomed 30-somethings, I could see that they took good care of themselves. But something was missing. They seemed pleasant enough. They smiled. They greeted me cordially. However, behind this façade, something was bothering them. I could feel that sense of urgency ready to burst through. I began the conversation.

"Very nice to meet you, Mr. & Ms. Halpern."

"The pleasure is ours," Izzie said.

"What can I do for you, Ms. Halpern? Are you the patient or is it your husband?"

Izzie and Allen looked at one another briefly, unsure of who should start talking. Allen then took the reins and answered the questions.

"It's actually both of us. You could say we're both patients, in different ways. Please call me Allen and my wife Izzie. We prefer it that way."

"Okay."

Allen began speaking.

"For the past several years, things have become a bit unraveled, you could say. I've been snoring more, which has caused a rift in our relationship. My wife can't sleep with my loud snoring. I don't notice it that much, although I'm tired as ever the following day. So, maybe there is some larger issue. But I'm sure that I don't have sleep apnea, like the rest of my friends. I'm in perfect shape. Well, almost."

Allen chuckled a bit, but I recognized that he thought he was fitter than most, which he was. He then went on to discuss a brawl in which he had recently been involved at a local bar. Apparently, Allen was ordering a drink when, out of nowhere, one of the patrons came up to him and called him a racial slur. This racist then told Allen to go to China where the coronavirus originated. A fight then ensued in which the assailant fractured Allen's nose. Allen also relayed that, although he had never realized that he snored before his fight at the bar, others had told him as much. The snoring and his fatigue just worsened after that incident.

Allen and Izzie were both silent as they looked at me for some recognition and insight. Their gaze suggested that they wanted me to provide them with a magic elixir that would solve their problems, so they could return to their blissful marriage. Isn't that what everyone desires? A quick solution to the problem. But, treatment for a medical condition creates new issues that often pose their own problems. Every treatment has side effects that must be weighed against one another. Each individual's treatment is different, and there is no single approach to the problem.

I continued my discussion with the couple.

"I'm sorry that happened to you. But based on what I'm hearing, it does appear that you both have sleep conditions that need to be addressed and treated. Allen, your problem is probably a form of sleep-disordered breathing, of which obstructive sleep apnea is a type. I would guess that it was probably exacerbated by the incident at the bar, given that your nasal passage might be obstructed after the nasal fracture. Izzie, your issue is that of an environmental sleep disorder, meaning that it is brought upon by an external source, namely Allen's snoring. So, once we remedy his problem, your sleep disorder should resolve, although that's not always the case.

Izzie suddenly became animated and began to tell the story she had probably wanted to tell someone for quite some time. She began her narrative.

"Initially, I tried to dismiss Allen's snoring. It wasn't 'that bad,' I thought. My other girlfriends had experienced something much worse, as they told me during our conversations. But Allen's snoring became worse, and much worse, in no time. It wasn't even a typical snore. It sounded as if air were trying to squeeze through a small ravine: a crescendo followed by a decrescendo and then a brief pause before it all began again. It was a cacophony."

Allen snarked a bit at this, but Izzie wasn't going to give up on her tirade. I prodded her on. I needed to see where she stood on this issue and how severe the problem was for her.

"Please continue, Izzie."

"Thanks, doctor. I really need to get this off my chest. Well, although I hadn't anticipated this snoring, we began sleeping in different rooms. But, no matter what I did, I could still hear Allen's snoring, obviously not as loudly, but loudly enough to prevent me from going to sleep at a timely hour. Customized ear plugs didn't work. A white noise machine barely made a dent. Smothering my ears with pillows was of no use. It's literally killing me a little bit each night. I absolutely cannot take it anymore."

She turned to Allen.

"Either you fix this problem, or I want a separation."

They looked awkwardly at one another, unsure of what to say next. I wasn't a marriage counselor, but I have often seen sleep disorders cause such rifts in relationships that divorces and separations become real possibilities. Then, Allen chimed in and deflected.

"You think I have sleep breathing, or whatever you called it, doctor?"

"Yes, I do. It's called sleep-disordered breathing, and contrary to what people think, about 20% of people with this disorder are actually thin, in good shape, and otherwise healthy, such as yourself. Obstructive sleep apnea, a form of sleep-disordered breathing, is either a complete or partial collapse of the airway and results in awakenings throughout the night. You may awake from these, or have arousals where your 'brain wakes up,' but you don't necessarily remember it. These repeated awakenings can cause all sorts of problems, some of which bring you to the clinic, like snoring and excessive daytime sleepiness. However, other effects of this problem include high blood pressure, heart issues, and headaches, among others."

Allen and Izzie looked incredulous, like I had told them a secret that had been hidden from them. Then Allen started.

"This could be serious, then? But, why me? I thought everyone with this problem was heavier than me. At least, some of my friends who have this problem have those characteristics. Are you really sure that I have this disorder?"

"Obviously, I can't be certain unless we do a polysomnogram, or sleep study. But you do meet the characteristics of those with this condition. Thin individuals with this condition have craniofacial structures like you do. They may also have a deviated nasal septum. I'll do a physical exam to verify this. But the good news is that those with a thin habitus tend to have a milder form of the disease."

"Well, that doesn't make me feel any better."

"I feel you. But, let me first conduct an exam and see where this leads us."

I asked Allen to open his mouth and flashed a light there. As I had surmised, Allen's airway was narrowed. His palate had a high arch and was constricted. Furthermore, I assessed his nasal passages via an otoscope, and, as I had guessed, he had a severe deviation of his septum, likely from the injury to his nose during that bar brawl.

"Now that I had a chance to look at your airway, I do think you have a high probability of having a form of sleep-disordered breathing. As I said before, we have to verify this with a sleep study, meaning you'll come here to the lab and sleep for the night. We'll have all sorts of electrodes attached to you, and a nasal oral sensor to see if you have any breathing events."

Allen was registering this, and Izzie was looking at him to gauge his response.

"Okay. That doesn't sound so bad. I think I can sleep through all that. I fall asleep pretty quickly but then wake up through the night."

"He'll have no problem falling asleep," Izzie said, laughing. "I'm the one who bears the brunt of the problem."

"Yes, let's address your problem, Izzie. As I said, once Allen's problem is treated, your insomnia should improve or resolve. However, your brain may have become so used to the snoring that, at least for a bit, you may have problems sleeping due to the absence of the snoring. You could use a sound machine for a brief period if you experience that."

"Trust me, doctor. That will never happen. I will never miss Allen's snoring. Never."

She emphasized her "never" several times to suggest that this was a nightly hell for her.

"Okay, I get it, Izzie," Allen said before turning to me again. "But, what is the treatment for this? I don't want to wear one of those strange devices on my face. CPAP, right? I simply refuse to do so."

"Like I said, let's do the sleep study and see what that shows. Depending on the severity of your sleep-disordered breathing—and that is presuming that you have the disorder—you may just require an oral appliance, a specialized pillow, or something of the sort to prevent you from lying on your back, or surgery to fix your deviated septum. So, yes, you may not have to resort to continuous positive airway pressure, or CPAP, although that remains the most effective treatment for this condition."

"I guess I can deal with the other options. I'm open to the sleep study. I'm hoping you're wrong, doctor, but I get the importance of knowing whether I have the condition."

It was now Izzie's turn. I could see her smiling mischievously, as if she had tricked her husband and was getting what she wanted all this time. Allen turned to her and asked her opinion.

"What do you think, babe?"

"It all sounds great to me. Like the doctor said, if you have sleep-disordered breathing, we have to address it one way or another. Doing nothing is not an option. Your blood pressure and marriage are teetering on the edge. Didn't your family doctor say that you may have to consider medications for your hypertension?"

"Yes, I guess he did. So, doctor, if I understand you correctly, treating my presumed breathing issue can potentially help with my elevated blood pressure, correct?"

I nodded. "Yes, you're absolutely right. Research has confirmed this, again and again. You'll get the greatest benefit with CPAP, of course, but the other treatment options are effective, too."

"Good to know. So, what's causing my insomnia in the middle of the night? Is it my presumed apnea?"

"Yes, probably. There is a high correlation between those who have obstructive sleep apnea and insomnia. The reason is that the brain registers the life-threating nature of the breathing cessation or decreased airflow and awakens you. You're probably not aware of most of these events, but there are some that consciously awaken you and then you're unable to return to sleep."

"That's exactly it. I don't know what's waking me up, but sometimes it's a loud snoring. And, then I'm up and lying in bed until I fall asleep again."

"If that happens to you and you can't return to sleep in 20 minutes, please leave the bedroom and go to the living room. Read a magazine or a book under dim lights and then return to bed when you're sleepy again. You don't want to reinforce your insomnia. This is called stimulus restriction. We want to sever the bad things that are associated with your insomnia. In this case, it's your bed and bedroom environment."

"That just makes me anxious, and I keep looking at the clock, thinking that I won't get enough sleep and won't be productive at work. At times, I think I can even get fired for being a slacker."

"There are two things that are problematic here. Looking at the clock will only make you more anxious, so please place the clock somewhere away from you, so that you're unable to look at it. Second, your idea about not being productive at work is a little skewed. Yes, you may be less productive at work and not function to your full capacity, but it's not a catastrophe. You'll get on and do just fine. Your work may not be optimal, but that's okay. We'll correct it in due time. From what you've told me, most days you're doing fine. It's the occasional episodes of insomnia that you're remembering. That's perfectly normal. As humans, we tend to catastrophize events that pose a problem for us, and, more importantly, we don't remember the episodes of insomnia that we didn't have—just the ones that trouble us. However, if you were to calculate the bad and good days of sleep, I'd venture to say that you've had more good than bad."

"Yeah, I'd probably agree with that. It's just that when I have a bad night of sleep—severe insomnia—I tend to ruminate about it. It ruins my entire day."

"Exactly. That's the effect of catastrophizing, making things bigger than they actually are and allowing them to take over your life. I get it. To a certain extent, we all do that. They key is to realize that you have control over this and it's not something that'll ruin your life. In fact, it's this phantom catastrophizing that will destroy you; your thoughts are powerful. Disengage from them. You are the one that's conjuring them. Without you, they'd be nothing."

"I never thought about it that way. I guess I've been creating this catastrophe for myself."

"The first step is to recognize it, and then you have to do something about it."

Izzie then began to question me.

"Let's say that Allen is diagnosed with sleep-disordered breathing and decides to use CPAP. Won't that machine, itself, prevent him from going to sleep? Aren't we just perpetuating his insomnia?"

Allen was forcefully nodding his head, in agreement with Izzie. I could tell that the last thing that he wanted to use was CPAP.

"Yes, that could be a possibility. But, if the breathing is preventing him from returning to sleep, then we may need to fix that. As I said, CPAP may not be the best option for Allen, assuming that he even has that condition. We can experiment with an oral appliance and positional techniques, depending on the severity of the condition. Or, we can focus on some cognitive behavioral techniques, some of which I touched upon, to tackle the insomnia. Let's say the condition is bad enough that CPAP may be warranted. We can then focus on desensitization therapy to help Allen get used to the mask by allowing him to place the mask on his face when he is awake. He can then use CPAP incrementally each night, first for 1 hour, then for 3 to 4 hours each night. Finally, he will use it for the entire night. If he still cannot use it, then a trial of sleep medication for the first month may be an option. Please let me reiterate, though: this all depends on the severity of Allen's condition, if he is diagnosed with sleep-disordered breathing."

Allen then began to speak.

"I get it. Let's do the sleep study and see what it shows. Now that I understand the diagnosis and some of the treatments for the condition, I'm more amenable to the entire process. Let's do it."

I could see the optimism in his face and demeanor.

Izzie was smiling, too.

Then they both clasped hands and left my office, resigned to whatever the future held for them.

☾

Sleep Pearls

As Allen's narrative suggests, not every insomnia is created equally. In his case, he had a history and physical examination that were compatible with a very serious medical condition called sleep-disordered breathing that was causing him to awaken when sleeping. It is important to recognize that medical issues can complicate insomnia and, once that particular condition is treated, then the insomnia can potentially resolve.

In Izzie's case, her sleep was affected by an external interruption, namely Allen's egregious snoring. One must be mindful of external interruptions like pain, noise, light, and some illnesses and medications that can be treated separately so that insomnia can resolve on its own. Again, be mindful of the fact that not all insomnia is the same and cannot be treated generically.

Jeremy

Nocturnal Panic Disorder and
Visualization Therapy

A T 4 A.M., JEREMY AWAKENS IN HIS VERY SPACIOUS AND minimalist Toy Factory loft near the southern edge of the Arts district in Downtown Los Angeles. The year is 2007. The once dilapidated city is undergoing a burgeoning—a renaissance, one might even say. He is at the heart of it. As the owner and Michelin-starred chef of a hip restaurant across from his loft, this 48-year-old successful entrepreneur has brought the food scene to this once-ensconced and forgotten neighborhood of Los Angeles. He should be proud. He should have no worries. He is successful, intelligent, and a maverick in his profession.

One night, however, he awakens suddenly. He looks at his alarm clock on the nightstand. It's 12:30 a.m. His heart is beating more than 120 beats per minute. His breathing is a little too fast and shallow. What could be causing this? Jeremy is as healthy as they come. He has no known medical conditions. He has not undergone any surgeries. He's the perfect specimen.

He looks at himself in the mirror. He doesn't recognize himself. Someone is watching him. He feels that he is looking at himself from an angle where he remains unrecognizable. He is hyperventilating. Jeremy feels that he is going to die. So, this is how it all ends, he thinks. His entire life has come down to this one moment. Although successful, he has no one. He thinks about his short relationship with Velouria, the Czech-born model he had been dating for the past 6 months. Those moments constituted the best months of his life. He can feel the waters of the Aegean Sea on the cruise they last took together to Santorini. He can feel their embrace, the way she made him feel safe in her arms. In those moments, with her at his side, he felt invincible. How could be so stupid and break off their relationship, just because he thought that she had flirted with another guy at the restaurant? It was mere jealousy, without any valid reasoning or justification. He knew that now, but it was too late. He had severed the relationship, coldly and cruelly, with a perfunctory text he had not thought twice about. Not to mention, the text was capitalized: DON'T CALL OR TEXT ME AGAIN. I DON'T WANT ANYTHING TO DO WITH YOU. LEAVE ME ALONE.

In these moments where he felt like he was dying, he realized that only Velouria could save him. He imagined her small arms that could lift his 6-foot-2-inch, 180-pound frame. He imagined himself and Velouria hovering above the ground together, directing the wind. His heart rate slowed. He was breathing more slowly too. He now felt that he could actually live to see Velouria.

Jeremy had read about panic attacks. Was this what he was experiencing? Jeremy came to see me for an evaluation to get to the bottom of it. He relayed what had prompted him to come.

"I'm a mess. I don't know what has happened to me in the last few weeks, but I'm actually afraid of sleeping. It actually makes me more tired. I would rather just stay awake than feel the hell that I experience every night when I attempt to sleep. I can't go on like this. I really need your help."

He described what he thought were panic attacks and I took it all in. Here was a successful entrepreneur, a chef, who once exuded confidence but was now utterly distraught. He looked haggard, his tousled, wavy hair jutting in all directions. There was swelling under his eyes, dark circles that revealed the vacuous space in which he now found himself.

"Is this the first time you've had panic attacks?" I asked.

"Yes, that was the first horrific one, but, since then, just thinking about it brings back that specific memory and other panic attacks that don't last as long. However, I anticipate them and can't sleep. It seems that the one panic attack started everything, and it's just kept everything going. In French, it's called 'cercle vicieux,' a vicious circle," he responded.

"It's a vicious circle, alright. Are you French?"

"Yes, I'm originally from France, although I've been in the United States for about 30 years now. I consider America home, although I return to France quite often.

"What part of France are you from?

"I was born in a small village that no one's heard of called Ville-franche-sur-Mer in Provence. It's spectacularly beautiful. As an adolescent and in the summer, I would often spend lazy afternoons enjoying that cool ocean breeze while sipping my coffee. I would just stare into that water and imagine myself out there swimming, free and without any worries. There's a vastness in the ocean that makes me feel so invincible and free. The town has a small 14th-century chapel with mystical frescoes painted by Jean Cocteau, the French novelist and film director, who spent his summers there. It's really something. You should experience it for yourself. You won't be disappointed."

"The way you're describing it, I want to be there now. It sounds like you have a close bond with that town."

"I do, and whenever I go to Paris, I manage to make a quick stop there, although I have no family there now. My parents have passed away and my aunts and uncles are scattered throughout Europe. I don't have much contact with them anymore."

I could tell that Jeremy had become guarded, and didn't want to discuss his family tree any further. I wasn't a psychiatrist, so I wasn't going to extend this thread.

"I know we've veered off topic a bit, so tell me about these panic attacks.

"Well, the first one just occurred suddenly. I woke up from sleep one night, my heart was racing, I couldn't breathe, and I thought I would pass out."

"Did you pass out?"

"No, I didn't. My heart was beating so rapidly, I was hyperventilating, and I thought that I would eventually faint, but, thankfully, I didn't."

"What did you do when this was occurring?"

"I was just pacing up and down my loft, not knowing what to do. I smoked a cigarette to help me relax, but it actually made everything worse. My heart was beating faster. I threw it out after a few puffs. I eventually took 1 mg of Ativan my primary care doctor had prescribed for me during long airplane flights. I have acrophobia and tend to get a bit anxious up in the air. I've been really trying not to take these anymore. But that was the only thing I could think of when this panic attack was occurring. I tried to find a paper bag to blow into, but I didn't have any. And, then, with the Ativan, I felt sleepy again, and thankfully dozed off until the morning. But I really did think I was going to die. My heart was racing that fast!"

"Let me guess. The problem now is that, every time you sleep, you recall the first panic attack you had and you think this will happen again. And, then, these intrusive thoughts won't allow you to sleep, right?"

"That's exactly right. You nailed it. Based on the way you're describing it, I guess I'm not the only one who has experienced this."

"You're certainly not, but that's a good thing, because we now have ways to deal with panic attacks that arise from sleep and methods to improve your sleep. But, let me ask you, when did this panic attack occur? Was it during the first half of the night or the latter half?"

"If I recall correctly, I went to bed fairly early that night, at least early for me. It was about 11:30 p.m. and I was super tired. I think it took me less than 10 minutes to fall asleep. But then I woke up about an hour later and looked at the alarm clock, which registered half past midnight. Why do you ask?"

"The timing for a nocturnal panic attack fits your scenario, which usually occurs in the first 90 minutes of sleep. If it had occurred later at night, we'd be concerned about a nightmare that prompted all of this, for which we'd use a different treatment option."

"Yeah, it was definitely not a nightmare, because I wasn't dreaming of anything. It just came out of the blue."

"Yes, so a nocturnal panic attack sounds right. Now, what do we do with that? As with many drugs, taking Ativan every night and building both a psychological and physical dependence on it is not ideal in the long run. In fact, if you become dependent on Ativan and quickly withdraw from it, you can have a seizure. You may experience some cognitive impairment with it, especially when you begin to age, so I'd like to move away from taking that medication."

"Man! I didn't know that. I certainly don't want to continue taking it if I have a choice."

"Doesn't it also make you tired?"

"I'm not sure anymore. Although I sleep, I feel like I'm not rested enough. This panic thing has turned into a monster that I can't seem to slay. I really need some treatment options that don't involve medication.

"We'll work on this with a few techniques. The first will be the tried-and-true visualization therapy, which I've had a great deal of success with, not only with regard to panic attacks but other diagnoses, as well."

"What is that?"

"Just like it sounds. When you feel that you're undergoing an attack or if you want to prevent one, focus on calming and relaxing images, things that you've enjoyed in the past and places where you've felt the most comfortable.

"Like the town that I grew up in? Sitting on the beach, next to the ocean, and drinking coffee is definitely something that relaxes me."

"Exactly. You couldn't have picked a better image. The way you describe that town is perfect. Now, in addition to visualizing, try to notice as many sensory details from that town as you can recall, like the colors of the sky and the ocean, the sounds you hear, and the briny smell of the sea. Take this all in, as if you were there. Not only will this visualization transport you there—the mind is a powerful thing—but it will also distract you from the panic and anxiety that you are experiencing at the moment. Listening to sounds of the ocean on your phone—there are many apps that simulate calming noises—may also work in conjunction with this visualization.

"I can definitely do that. I can even picture it now. It's one of my best memories."

"The visualization doesn't necessarily have to be of a location, either. It can be of a person you are close with or have had a great memory of, someone who can help you through one of your attacks. Are you single or married?"

"I'm single, but I just came out of a somewhat tumultuous relationship. I regret how I ended it with this woman I think I really loved. I know I was the one to blame for that disaster. She really brought out the best in me and I felt very safe in her arms. It's a weird thing to say, but she really was the stronger one in our relationship. Her name was Velouria, and I always think about her and it brings a smile to my face."

"Again, another powerful image that you can use whenever you feel these attacks. Feel her close to you, clasping you, and calming you. I'm sure that she feels the same about you."

"No, that part of things fell apart and is now over. I can never win her over after the way I broke it off. But I'm working that through with a therapist. It's been a long and winding road, for sure."

"Well, no need to dwell on the negative. Just think about those perfect moments you experienced together. Those memories can never be taken away from you. They're yours and they're etched deeply in your cortex. Use them to your advantage when you need them the most."

"You're right. Any other techniques that will help me sleep better?

"We're really dealing with your nocturnal panic attacks at this point, because once we sever that, your sleep should normalize. A great breathing technique that can also help get you through these attacks is the 4-7-8 method. It was developed by Dr. Andrew Weil at The University of Arizona. It helps to increase the parasympathetic system and diminish the sympathetic, or fight-or-flight mode, system that is creating the panic attack."

"How does that work?"

"First, empty your lungs of air. Breathe in quietly through the nose for 4 seconds. Hold your breath for a count of 7 seconds. Then, exhale forcefully through your mouth, pursing the lips and making a whoosh sound, for 8 seconds. You can repeat this up to 4 times, until you feel relaxed again. If you can deploy this technique early on, you can interrupt the attack at its incipient stages before it veers out of control."

"That sounds great and pretty simple. I can definitely try this technique."

"There's also another technique, called progressive muscle relaxation, or PMR, that involves tensing and relaxing your major muscle groups. It's counterintuitive because the last thing you think of doing during these panic attacks is tensing your already tense muscles even more. But that is the beauty of this. When you tighten these muscles and release them, the release is that much greater and much more relaxing. We can try these techniques here.

Jeremy was focused. He attempted the 4-7-8 technique first, but he did the process too quickly. I told him to slow down because the ratio of time spent exhaling or inhaling was crucial. I told him that he could speed or slow down the process as long as the ratio remained the same. But, at its basic level, the 4-7-8 sequence was the most efficient. To switch up the ratio would not work. So, Jeremy tried the technique again and immediately felt the effect. He could feel his heart rate and breathing slow.

"Wow. How did that happen? Why am I so relaxed now?"

I laughed, because Jeremy was now experiencing the benefits of this very simple, yet effective, technique.

"Scientifically, this response is activated by the vagus nerve, which is a parasympathetic nerve. It's like a brake that puts a stop to the sympathetic system, or the fight-or-flight mode. In our caveman days, the fight-or-flight response was especially helpful when we would have to flee predators. However, in this modern age, we don't need that system when we're sleeping peacefully in bed and have no reason to fight or flee from anyone."

"That makes sense. I shouldn't be feeling anxious. I'm super grateful for all the success that has followed me and there shouldn't be a reason for this anxiety. Except, perhaps, my past relationship with Velouria. But I'm working through this."

"Your initial panic attack probably had nothing to do with her, but now the original panic attack is fueling all the other attacks."

"I agree with that."

"The 4-7-8 technique is also valuable because it increases your heart rate variability, meaning that when you exhale, your heart rate decreases and when you inhale, your heart rate increases. The greater the difference between these two rates, the more effective the heart is in pumping the blood to your various organs and tissues. A lower heart rate variability is observed in several cardiovascular and respiratory diseases, such as hypertension and COPD, which demonstrates this abnormal adaptability. So, heart rate variability is a good thing."

"I didn't even know any of this. These are powerful. Thank you."

"You're welcome, but all of this needs to be practiced during the day. The more adept you are at this, the less of a chance there is that your panic attack will get out of control. That's why practicing is so important. It's like a play. You don't want to learn your lines while on stage. You want to nail them down before you go on stage."

"Should I still be taking Ativan?

"That's a good question. You don't necessarily have to take it. Our goal for you is to eventually discontinue this medication. However, have it on hand just in case your panic attack becomes full-blown. A rescue medication can be a great idea. Just knowing that you have something on hand allays your anxiety to a significant degree. Keep it by your bedside. Recognize that although you probably won't use it, it's there if you need it. Kind of like your memories."

"Perfect. I'm really looking forward to sleeping tonight. It's been at least a few weeks since I've slept so well."

"But don't create expectations for yourself. Don't fall into that trap. See how the night proceeds. Having a goal of sleeping well can create its own anxiety. Let the chips fall where they may. I'll follow up with you in a couple of weeks to see how things are progressing."

With this thought, Jeremy thanked me and exited the doors of the sleep clinic. Although I couldn't see his face, his posture was more erect, and his gait was more firm and unyielding. I knew his sleep and anxiety would improve with time. In his mind, at least, he had access to Villefranche-sur-Mer and Velouria, anytime, anywhere.

☾ Sleep Pearls

As Jeremy's case demonstrates, visualization therapy is an immensely powerful tool that is underappreciated and underutilized for insomnia rooted in anxiety. The key to this technique is to "see" and project yourself into an environment or with people who make you feel safe. You can use your various other senses to add depth and vibrancy to these images, feelings, and ideas to make them come to life. Such visualizations can be used very effectively with the 4-7-8 breathing technique that will activate your parasympathetic system and effectively place your body in a state of rest and relaxation. Like Jeremy, find your own Velouria or Villefranche-sur-Mer and transport yourself to a personal Shangri-la so you can sleep better.

Mary

Advanced Sleep Phase Syndrome and Early Morning Insomnia

Note to readers: In duplicitous fashion, and in order to make this case unique, I have fashioned myself as Mr. Sandman. These are not meant to be authentic letters; rather, they have been fictitiously used to entertain while teaching you about advanced sleep phase syndrome. Also, they are meant to suggest the ubiquity of advice columns about sleep and how they should be vetted to ensure that the solution is rooted in science.

Dear Mr. Sandman,

I've really enjoyed your advice column over the years. I've learned so much from the advice you've given to those insomniac readers of yours. You really are something! I mean that. You sprinkle that magic sand in their eyes, so they can sleep deeper and more peacefully, and dream a little dream. I've read your stories from afar, never having the courage to tell my own. I think it's now time to delve into my own problem and pester you with it. Oh, I hope you can help me,

Mr. Sandman. I know that's not your real name, but you are *my* Sandman. I'm a 75-year-old woman from Seattle, Washington, who has
been having this problem now for almost 20 years. Twenty *long* years,
I should add. I'm afraid it's getting a little worse each night, too. While
most people my age have trouble falling asleep, I have the opposite
problem. I actually want to stay up, and yet I can't! Isn't that the most
ludicrous thing you've heard? But, then, when I wake up too early,
I can't go back to sleep. It's horrible! So, I guess I have insomnia, or
maybe not? You tell me. My husband Harold says I need to just stay up
a little longer and then my body would just get used to it. Like it's that
easy. But, cross my heart, I just can't do it. My Harold even told me
that I'm just doing this to spite him because I can't stand the neighbors
he plays bridge with, every other night. I don't necessarily like Betty,
but I don't despise her, either. "Heavens to Betsy!" I told him. "How can
you say such a thing?" Of course, I don't go to sleep out of spite. I just
can't stay up. It's like Mr. Sandman sprinkles that sand of his in my
eyes a bit too early. He laughed at this. He facetiously said that you, Mr.
Sandman, don't exist. But I know you exist, Mr. Sandman. Your advice
column is wonderful. Harold doesn't get it. I'm afraid it's causing a rift
in our relationship. We've been married for 50 blissful years, so I don't
want my sleep disturbance to ruin it all. I'm hopeful that you can help
me through this ordeal. Don't put sand in my eyes too early, okay? I
have faith in you.

My best regards,
Sleeping (Too Early) in Seattle

Dear Sleeping (Too Early) in Seattle,

Things are not lost. I surmise that you and Harold still have many
blissful golden years ahead of you. The rain and downcast sky may
reign over your city now, but I am forecasting continued blue sky and

golden sunshine for you both. You are right, though. You don't have a classic form of insomnia. It sounds to me like your circadian rhythm is a little advanced compared to Harold's and your neighbors', which is not necessarily a bad thing. But, in your case, it just doesn't jive with everybody's schedule, and that's a shame. But the good news is, we can easily fix this. I'm afraid that Seattle is not really helping your situation, either. But please don't fret, Sleeping in Seattle. If you desire that the Sandman sprinkle sand in your eyes a little later, your solution is to get some sunlight in your eyes a couple of hours before you sleep. Because you live in Seattle and you don't get sunlight very often, you'll need a lightbox. That is, unless you're experiencing those blue skies and beautiful golden rays of sunshine Seattle is known for in those few blissful months of summer. It's a little complicated to explain here, but please see a sleep specialist if you have the inclination. They'll set you on the right path with a good sleep regimen, so you can play bridge with Harold and your neighbors—that is, if you really want to. You shouldn't be forced to do something that you don't want to do. Ever. That's the best advice I can offer you.

Sleep a little sleep and dream a little dream,
Mr. Sandman

Dear Mr. Sandman,

I know that you suggested I see a doctor for my sleep problem, but you're the best doctor I know. I think I'll stick with you, if you don't mind. I tried the lightbox, but I guess I forgot to ask you when to use it. I usually start to feel sleepy around 7 p.m. and can probably sleep then. I try to stay up as much as I can, but you tend to sprinkle that sand in my eyes at around 7:30 p.m., just like clockwork. I'm gone then, to peaceful slumber, while my Harold plays those card games with our neighbors, Betty and John. (Betty is a widow and John is a widower, but they are not romantically linked. What a shame! They'd be so good together.) It's mainly bridge they play, and they drink gin when playing it. Bridge is normally a four-person game, so you can imagine how guilty I feel when I can't stay up to play with them. I don't mean to badmouth Betty, but she can outdrink both Harold and John, although no one else sees it. They all have such a good time, while I'm sleeping. And, then, when I wake up at 4 a.m., I'm all alone. My dear Harold is still asleep, snoring. I nudge him softly. He then turns to his side and stops snoring. I don't want to go to our living room by myself, all alone, without Harold. I just stay in bed, looking at him, not able to sleep. Occasionally, I go outside and tend to my little garden that I'm slowly cultivating. It's not so difficult to see the garden grow so beautifully here in Seattle, with the abundance of all that rain. Harold gets up at 9 a.m., feeling refreshed, while I look like an absolute zombie. I can't compete with that Betty, when I look so haggard, while she looks like she just stepped out of the hair salon, hair just right and a nice-looking lipstick to boot. I just want to be in their circle to see what the fuss is all about. Mr. Sandman, please tell me what to do.

Best,
Still Sleeping (Too Early) in Seattle

Sleeping (Too Early) in Seattle,

I'm flattered that you think of me as the best doctor to solve your sleep problem. For the sake of transparency, I *am* a board-certified sleep physician. But I usually don't correspond in this column, back-and-forth to my readers. Because I imagine a great deal of people, especially those who are getting older, have this problem, I'll oblige you. (Something tells me that you're still young at heart, though.) Your 24-hour body clock, which is located inside your brain, behind your eyes, makes you sleepy between the hours of 7 to 8 p.m. and alert as early as 3 a.m., if I understand you correctly. By contrast, the body clock of most adults (like your dear Harold) makes them feel sleepy between the hours of 11 p.m. to 1 a.m., and alert at other times (6 to 9 p.m. and 8 to 11 a.m.). About 1% of middle aged to older people experience this advance phase sleep disorder, which can result in insomnia in the early morning and daytime sleepiness and fatigue, as well as increasing the risk of depression. Count yourself one of the unique few! What we have to do is to realign your body clock so that it resembles that of Harold and your neighbors. How will we do this? As I've explained before, you need a lightbox to use in the evening, which, apparently, you have been. However, your timing may be off. If you're feeling sleepy at 7:30 p.m., you should be using the light box for at least an hour (preferably 2) before that time. In your case, that would be 5:30 p.m. Now, that doesn't mean that you have to be staring at it for those 2 hours (that's ridiculous and I wouldn't subject you to that). But please situate the box in a place where the light could shine indirectly into your eyes, on top of a computer maybe or a small television set. It's your choice. But turn the device off a half-hour before bed. You should also get an eye exam first and make sure that you don't have cataracts or macular degeneration before using the light box; ultraviolet rays and shorter wavelength blue light can contribute to those conditions and worsen them. You may just need to use this light box every night for a week, or you may need several weeks. It depends on your reaction to the light.

Although the light box is the best solution to your problem, I would also recommend that you take melatonin in the early morning hours; that could further delay your rhythm and reset your body clock. Our objective is to delay your sleep, which basically means allowing yourself to sleep later, so you can play bridge with your friends. With regard to melatonin, you can do one of two things. One option is to take a 2-mg slow-release melatonin tablet close to your new bedtime. The other option is to take a small dose (0.5 mg) of melatonin when you wake up at 4 a.m. The second option may make you a little groggy at first, but your body will acclimate to this over time until you get your rhythm just right. As you can see, you will be delaying your bedtime by about 30 minutes each night until you get a time that best suits your needs. As such, you will also be delaying the exposure of your light box and intake of melatonin over the next few weeks. It may seem a little too much at first, but you'll get the hang of it in no time. (Your questions make me think that you're pretty adept and smart.) Now go out and delay your rhythm. There's no better time than today.

Carpe noctem: enjoy the night's pleasures,
Mr. Sandman

Mr. Sandman,

Thank you! Thank you! Thank you! I don't know how to repay you. I know it's been a while since I last wrote to you, but I've been busy practicing what you taught me. It was a little difficult at first, getting everything just right. I had to get the light box aligned perfectly, so that it was hitting my eyes. I don't want to be a victim of cataracts and macular degeneration from using the light box. But wouldn't you know it? The light made me so much more alert at night. At first, it was just a little, but the more I used it, the more energetic I became at night. I had been trying to hide the light box from Harold (he doesn't need to know about our secret), but he stumbled upon it one night while I was using it. "What is that, a magic contraption of some sort?" I laughed and told him that it was a genie, imprisoned in a box. I was trying to free it, so that it could make my wish come true. "Ha! Ha!" he remarked. "So, *what* is your wish?" I didn't even flinch. "To be able to sit and play with you, dear. I don't want to miss out on the fun that you and our neighbors have together." He then came and hugged me.

Gradually, I began to extend my sleep time and take my melatonin a little later each night. Harold and the neighbors play bridge at 9 p.m. each night and it lasts about 2 hours. Finally, about 6 weeks after I began using the melatonin and light box, I felt that I was ready to stay up and play that game of theirs. I remember walking up to that table, which is situated outside our porch. John was very hospitable and hugged me, saying how much he would enjoy if I joined them. Of course, I would join them and play this game of theirs. But I could tell that Betty wasn't happy with this. "What a hoot!" she said. "Finally, Mary can join us! I had never seen this day coming." Her remark, although good-natured, had tinges of sarcasm and mockery. I dismissed it. I'd tried to play nicely with her and this is how I was treated. This is what I was waiting for these 6 months: to show her that I am up to the challenge, that she can't steal Harold from me.

It was then that I grabbed Harold by the arms, brought his face close to mine, and kissed him. All the while, Betty's gaze was transfixed on us. It was all worth it—the light box, the melatonin, and the daily regimen.

Grateful,
Sleeping (Peacefully) in Seattle

☾

Sleep Pearls

Advanced sleep phase syndrome (ASPS), the polar opposite of delayed sleep phase syndrome—remember Savannah?—is seldom seen in the sleep clinic, not because it is less prevalent or less problematic but because those suffering from it either think this sleep disorder is innate or that there is not much that can be done about it. However, as Mary's case demonstrates, this syndrome mimics insomnia and can affect one's lifestyle and relationships. However, it can be successfully treated. Treatment consists of melatonin intake after early morning awakenings or upon finally arising in the morning. Bright light therapy, in the form of a light box, can be administered for 2 hours prior to your usual sleep time.

If you're waking up too early and are not able to return to sleep, always consider ASPS in addition to the classical diagnosis of insomnia. The two may coexist. If they do coexist, the advanced phase may need to be treated first before the insomnia is tackled.

Case 8

Bruce

Sleep on a Shift Schedule

B RUCE ARRIVED AT MY OFFICE IN A FEVERISH STATE. He was a 35-year-old nurse who had recently been placed on leave from his job because of his sleepiness. He had been working a night shift, something that he had not done before; something disastrous had occurred during this shift, which is the reason he had come to see me. His sleep time was fairly normal—more a morning lark than a night owl—but nothing too extreme. Generally, he would awaken at 6 a.m. and retire to bed at 11 p.m., which was actually an ideal bedtime schedule for him. However, in the past several years, his sleep had become tempered when he entered nursing school and, more recently, with the start of his night shift at the hospital. Bruce was somewhat reticent to initiate the dialogue, so I started."

"What can I do for you, Mr. Hawthorne?"

"Call me Bruce, please. Recently, there has been so much going on that I feel my life is helter-skelter. I had such a normal schedule, well fairly normal, and now I feel I'm in a downward spiral."

Bruce said all these things very languidly, as if he'd been depleted of all energy. His tone indicated to me that he had already given up, that there was nothing anyone could do for him. He needed to be saved, and there was no messiah in sight.

"Well, can you tell me what has been happening?"

He went into the story of what had occurred in the hospital, the unfortunate incident with one of his patients, and how this had cost him his self-confidence, not to mention the agony and shame of essentially causing the patient significant pain and suffering before she improved. Because of his sleepiness during a graveyard shift at the hospital, Bruce had mistakenly miscalculated the amount of sodium to be placed in a patient's IV bag, and, as a result, the patient had sustained an acute neurological injury. Bruce had been placed on leave until he was able to acclimate to his shift-work schedules. He told me that he was grateful that the hospital had given him a second chance. I asked why the hospital had not given him the opportunity to just work day-shifts, so that he didn't have to resort to acclimating to a circadian rhythm that was out of alignment for him. Bruce said they had mentioned this, but he just felt that he would be taking the easy way out if he at least didn't try to adjust to the night-shift schedule. Also, it wasn't fair to the other nurses, who would pine for the morning shift. He was always good at everything he tried, so why had he not mastered this? he thought.

Bruce went on to talk about his sleep history. The pivotal point came about during nursing school, when he realized that he could never again sleep the way he used to. Sleep didn't feel natural anymore. It became something that he needed to get, not something that was a natural part of him. He was always grasping at it, to get more of it, but it would always elude him. He had thrown sleep off-kilter.

Immediately after nursing school, Bruce had enviably secured a job at a major teaching hospital in Los Angeles. The pay was great. The perks were fantastic. And the reputation of the hospital and the nursing staff was top-notch. He knew he had to alternate day and night shifts, working normal hours during the day but also working evening to morning hours when the need arose. However, he convinced himself that he was ready. His new title, and the confidence that came with it, made him feel he could handle anything. He would be wrong.

I began the conversation:

"Well, although I understand your frustration, the important thing is that your patient Bonny improved and is on the path to a normal recovery. Isn't that correct?"

"Yes, that's true, and thanks for putting a positive spin on this. But, truthfully, I love being a nurse, and, when I return to work, I know that I will have to work night shifts again. I don't think I can handle it. I'm here for some much-needed advice."

"Let's start with the basics. From what you told me earlier, your circadian rhythm is fairy-aligned. You go to bed at a normal time and wake up at a decent time, and, in total, obtain about 7 hours of sleep. Correct?"

"That's right."

"Well, working a night shift throws your natural rhythm out of alignment. Your natural urge is to sleep at night while, with this new routine, you're expected to stay awake. Some individuals are able to adapt to this fairly well, but most have to be retrained. It's not easy, but it can be done."

"So, how do I do this?"

"Let's start with the basics. You will inevitably get less sleep working a night shift. That's almost guaranteed and expected. The first step is to accept this fact and be content with it."

"Okay. This doesn't sound promising at all."

"It actually is, because part of dealing with shift work is to allow your brain to think of sleep in a different manner and to place it in a different context. Shift work is not natural. Our bodies have been made to sleep in certain way, both through chemicals and light, which are what we call *zeitgebers*, a German term that literally means 'time giver.' For our purposes, it means any environmental time cues, such as bodily chemicals, sunlight, alarm clocks, or social interactions that allow us to follow a 24-hour cycle. Light, and especially natural sunlight, is the most powerful cue we have at our disposal to allow us to modify our 24-hour cycle."

"That's interesting. I never knew that the light and all those other factors could affect my sleep so much."

"Definitely. So, let's start with light, the most potent zeitgeber; most of our treatment will be focused on this. It's summer now, so the sun sets at around 7:30 p.m. here in Los Angeles. When you went to work, did you wear sunglasses?"

"That's a strange question, but, yes, I usually did, like any other person who doesn't want that hot sun in their eyes."

Bruce chuckled, as if he didn't recognize the relevance of this question or how it fit into his problem. I could tell that although Bruce would be open to my suggestions, he was still a skeptic at heart.

"The reason I'm asking is that we have to reverse everything when you start a night shift. When you're going to work, and although the sun will set soon, it's essential that you treat this like you're beginning work, which you are. Drop those sunglasses and let the light in. You're tricking your hypothalamus into thinking that it's morning. Usually that part of the brain gets its information from a relay network that starts with the optic nerve receiving light into the eye."

"I never thought about it that way. That's clever that we can manipulate the brain to think that way."

"Yes, it is. The brain is extraordinary in what it can make us believe. During the summer, when you're driving to work to the hospital, you must make sure that you get adequate sunlight. Putting on your sunglasses is not the right approach because it blocks the light from entering your retina and sending that message to your brain to wake up. In the winter and even in California, you won't have the luxury of light in the evenings when you're driving to work. During these times, you should invest in a lightbox to simulate natural light, similar to what is used to treat seasonal affective disorder."

"I get it. It's like I'm driving to work in the morning, right?"

"Exactly. Now, the same logic must be followed when you're driving from work to home. Now, you'll be doing the opposite because you want to simulate nighttime. That would be the time to wear your sunglasses. You would want to minimize any exposure to sunlight at that time."

"Okay. I can certainly do those things. What about the other zeitgebers you mentioned earlier?"

"Glad you remembered that. Yes, sunlight is the most powerful, but melatonin is also essential."

"I sort of know what melatonin is, but isn't that used for insomnia?"

"Actually, first and foremost, melatonin is essential in establishing our natural circadian rhythm. Yes, it can help with insomnia, but that is not its natural role. It's a hormone that is produced by the brain's pineal gland to regulate our circadian rhythm so that we can adapt to our natural sleep cycle and not have side effects like grogginess and sleepiness."

"Is there a particular time that I should take this for shift work?"

"Yes, this should be taken several hours before you plan to sleep. So, if you're leaving your shift at 7 a.m., I would take it at 5 a.m. I would take only 0.5 mg instead of the usual 3 mg the stores normally sell. Remember, you are really using this to regulate your circadian rhythm, not for sleep, per se, although it will make you somewhat sleepy, too."

"Okay. Got that. What else can I do?"

"If you have rotating shifts, like morning, evening, and night shifts, ask your supervisor if they can schedule you in a clockwise rotation, meaning that your new shift should have a later start time than your earlier shift. The reason for this is that your body has a much easier time staying up later than going to bed earlier. That's the reason why flights to the east are much more grueling than those to the west. We have a mantra in the sleep world about this: west is best; east is a beast. When flying east, you battle the sleep beast."

"I hadn't heard that before, but, yeah, when I travel, I do find that trips to the east coast are much more taxing on me. It's really difficult for me to sleep in New York, for example, when I arrive there at 9 p.m. and am expected to fall asleep in a couple of hours, when it's early evening in my time zone."

"Exactly, Bruce. But you're not alone. It's our circadian rhythm that's dictating this."

I could tell that Bruce was absorbing this information, bit by bit, and was understanding how this fit into the larger picture of his sleepiness when he worked a night shift. His eyes were still distrustful of the information that I was providing him, but they were showing a hint of confidence. I continued with other suggestions.

"Also, if possible, take a 30- to 60-minute nap prior to reporting for a night shift. If that's not feasible, and, if allowed, take a 30-minute nap at work. Is that possible for you?"

"Well, I live alone, so taking a nap before work sounds like the best option. I guess I can also take a nap during my break at work. It'd be more difficult to do it then, but there's always my car. We have a nurse's lounge, but I can't fathom I could nap there with all the potential noise."

"Agreed. It has to be a quiet place, so that there is a possibility that you can sleep."

"I'm already anxious enough, so I can't allow any distractions because I know then that I *won't* be able to sleep."

Bruce emphasized the word "won't" as if he had calculated all the possibilities out there, especially the possibility that good sleep was out of reach for him now. I tried to steer him away from this catastrophic way of thinking that I've seen from my patients, time and time again.

"On another note, please try to keep a routine and schedule that doesn't change throughout the week or weekends. Obviously, your shifts will change throughout the week, but on those days that you work the same shift, try to keep a consistent schedule. Such a routine is basically telling your body to get used to this rhythm, to tell you when it's time to stay alert and when to sleep."

"Okay. But what am I supposed to do when my shifts change and I need to switch up my routine, if I have to transition from the evening shift, for example, to the night shift?"

The timbre of Bruce's voice was rising, as if I were giving him advice only to create more questions and obstacles for him.

"Great point, let's say that you are working the evening shift, which is from 5 p.m. to 1 a.m. You'd like to get a full 7 or 8 hours of sleep per night, or at least that's our hope. In such a scenario, you could sleep from 3 a.m. to 11 a.m. and then wake up to do whatever you needed until 5 p.m., when your evening shift would start. As I mentioned, if you feel like you could become sleepy again during your shift, take a 30-minute nap about an hour before you have to head to work."

"Okay. So, what about when I transition to the night shift?"

"So, let's say your night shift is 11 p.m. to 7 a.m. Do you have a couple days' notice before this switch?"

"Yes, I usually have about 2 to 3 days off before I make a transition from evening to night or night to day."

"Great. What we are trying to do here is to transition you from your evening shift routine to your night shift routine slowly, so that there won't be a stark break between the two. So, let's say you make this switch gradually over 3 days. On night one of the transition, you'd want to go to bed a couple of hours later while still getting your 8 hours of sleep. Instead of going to bed from 3 a.m. to 11 a.m., you would instead go to sleep from 5 a.m. to 1 p.m. On the second night, you'd shift that back another couple hours, and so on and so forth, until you're ready to work the night shift. Remember, it's always easier to go to sleep later than earlier. It's just the way our circadian rhythm is geared."

"That's good to know. I think I can do that. Now that I sort of know where I'm going with my sleep schedule, what about substances? I don't mean drugs, but things like nicotine and coffee. Yes, I know that I'm a nurse and should know better, but I still can't let go of my smoking. Will that affect anything?"

"Great point. Yes, chemicals are a big factor that should be considered whenever we're thinking of modifying our circadian rhythm. Anything that stimulates the brain while we plan to sleep or, on the other hand, stupefy it while we're trying to stay awake, is a problem."

"That's what I figured. I know that coffee is a vice that I can't seem to let go of while working in the unit. It's at the nurses' station and it's the easiest thing to drink while I'm about to fall asleep. Do I need to stop drinking it?"

"No, you need not be that extreme, especially if you enjoy coffee. In fact, a couple of cups of coffee earlier or in mid-shift is something that I recommend to my patients. However, timing is key. About 3 hours prior to your shift ending, you should definitely stop drinking it, because then you won't be able to sleep in the morning when you return from work. Same with nicotine. It's an alerting substance and smoking it closer to when you would go to bed will make sleep much more difficult. There are also a variety of nootropics—smart drugs that can boost brain performance—on the market that have been FDA-approved for shift work, such as Nuvigil, that you can take prior to your shift beginning. These don't have the same untoward side effects that amphetamines have. However, they can cause more insomnia that we can anticipate and headaches can be a concern."

"Maybe we can discuss the medication later. I'd like to see if I can solve this thing naturally without resorting to medication. Also, I don't like the idea of headaches."

"Of course, and that was my plan. I just wanted to let you know that, should you not improve significantly with these recommendations, we can always try nootropics."

"So do you think it's sustainable for me to work multiple night shifts in a row? Is there a recommended number of night shifts that my body could handle?"

"Yes, and I'm glad that you brought that up. In general, if you're working a 12-hour shift, you should limit work to 4 shifts in a row. No more than that. And, if possible, you should take more than 48 hours off after these shifts. Also, please avoid frequently rotating shifts. Our body has a more difficult time adapting to rotating shifts than it does to the same shift for the same amount of time."

Bruce was calculating all these schedules and shifts in his head. Could he really do this? he was probably thinking. What if he couldn't? Would he have to resort to working day-shifts only?

"Let me ask you another thing, Bruce. How peaceful is your home environment when you arrive home from the hospital?"

"It's totally quiet. I live alone, without any pets, so everything is super peaceful."

"That's good to know. If you had family members or friends living there, you'd want to make sure they stopped some of their noisy activities, like washing dishes, vacuuming, listening to music, and so forth, while you were trying to go to sleep. We often forget about environmental noise, but it can really impact the way we sleep."

"Yeah, I need to tune out everything. I'm especially sensitive to any external stimuli. You could say that's one of the reasons I'm single and live alone."

He chuckled when he said this, but I knew that the truth ran deeper than this. This topic was far beyond the scope of this visit.

"But, seriously, Bruce, you also need to have time for social activities and meeting with friends. Dealing with shift-work is not easy and if you don't have a support system, things can get messy very fast. Don't put in excessive overtime, either. That will just worsen the problem."

"Got it. Yeah, I was never very social, but am really good at giving orders. I need to work on my personality and delivery, that's for sure. This incident has taught me to be humble and forgiving of people. I really think this incident was a divine lesson, a divine hammer, to drive home the fact that people make mistakes, that I made a mistake, that I'm just as fallible as the next person."

"Take it one step at a time, but I think that you're on the right path. One last thing before we conclude our first session: if at any time you feel tired or sleepy after a night shift, make sure that you take a quick nap or find an alternative way home, like calling a friend or taking an Uber or Lyft. I've seen a lot of accidents occur over the years when a person has been too tired to drive home but does it anyway. In fact, getting poor sleep clouds one's judgment and, in some cases, is worse than driving under the influence. It's not worth endangering your life or the lives of others for an extra 30 minutes."

"I agree. I've always abided by that philosophy, so don't worry about that."

"When's your next shift at work?"

"It's in about 2 weeks."

"Okay. I want you to simulate the night-shift a couple of nights before you actually go to work. Give yourself a practice run and implement those things that we spoke out. Then, I want to see you back here in about 2 weeks."

"Will do. Thanks, again. I hope this works."

Bruce left the office a little lighter than he was when he came in. He opened the office door resolutely, turning the door knob with a good grip. I've come to learn that a strong grip is always a good sign of what's to come.

☾

Sleep Pearls

Shift work is a vexing problem for both individuals and for society. The safety of workers and those whom they care for, as Bruce's case demonstrates, is caught in such a nexus. High-profile disasters, such as the nuclear plant meltdown at Chernobyl in 1986 and the Exxon Valdez accident in 1989, have occurred in part thanks to work-related fatigue and carelessness. Luckily, treatment for this disorder is relatively simple and effective.

Preparing yourself for a night shift involves some planning. If you're tired or sleepy prior to a shift, a nap of 30 to 60 minutes can be effective, as can a nap in the workplace. Ensure that you obtain an adequate amount of light to work (via sunlight or a light box) and, conversely, wear sunglasses on your way from work to home. A small dose of melatonin 2 hours prior to when you usually sleep should also be used.

A note about Bruce: Although his acclimatization to his shift schedule was not as sudden or smooth as he initially assumed, with time and use of the strategies discussed, he was able to successfully work these shifts while remaining vigilant. For the days that he felt fatigued, he was prescribed Nuvigil to take prior to his night shift. He also tempered his personality and was able to establish camaraderie with his coworkers, which helped his mood and sleep.

Thao

Restless Leg Syndrome

THEY CAME IN TOGETHER, MOTHER AND SON. THAO was a 55-year-old Vietnamese woman. Vu, her 18-year-old son who had just graduated from high school, was enrolling in Princeton next year. You could see that Thao was so proud of her son. Her eyes were glimmering. She wanted to announce the fact that her son, American-born but without the advantages of other similarly situated students, had excelled and worked so hard over the past 4 years that he had now been accepted into one of the most prestigious universities in the world. It was the first thing she told me. Vu was a bit embarrassed by this statement and crouched a little, but he had grown accustomed to this gloating by his mom. "Mom," he said, "please stop it. It's so embarrassing." I interjected and added, "That's quite an accomplishment. You should be announcing this to everyone. Only about 5% of applicants are accepted to Princeton, right? That's very commendable." Vu acquiesced and nodded his headed without saying anything. I didn't want to belabor this point, so I just continued.

"What can I do for you, Ms. Tran?"

"My mom can't speak English that well," Vu started, "so I'm here to translate those sentences that she can't understand. Although, she can probably understand a lot more that she would like to think."

"Perfectly fine. I'm glad you accompanied her. What seems to be her sleep problem?"

Thao interjected at this point. "I can't sleep, doctor. It's so hard. It's hard when I lie down. I can't sleep."

Vu added. "Yeah, my mom has a difficult time going to sleep. She just lies there. I see how uncomfortable she is. My parents are divorced, so I often come into my mom's room to see how she is doing. And she's always awake, even at 2 a.m. I used to occasionally study late into the morning hours when I was applying to universities, and I would just see her so miserable. She would just lie there, looking up at the ceiling, and moving her legs a little. She would then get out of bed and start walking around the room, pacing back and forth. *Mệt mỏi.* I'm tired, she would say. So tired."

"Yes, doctor," Thao said. "I'm so tired all the time. I don't know why this is."

"We'll disentangle this," I said. "First, please tell me how long this has been occurring, and why you came to see me now?"

Vu started again.

"I began to see my mom really having this problem about 6 months ago when I started my senior year in high school. Initially, I thought she was becoming nervous because of my applying to schools. She has really sacrificed so much for me since we arrived here in the United States about a decade ago. She became so uprooted from her family, who wanted her stay in a small village in Hanoi. She was married there, and my parents immigrated here together. Well, it was too much for my father, so my parents eventually divorced. He returned to Hanoi. But my mom, because she knew that I would have opportunities here that I couldn't imagine in Vietnam, decided to stay here. It was really a struggle for her and I know that I won't ever be able to repay her. Part of the reason that I was accepted to Princeton was that drive she instilled in me from such a young age. I also wanted to repay her for all the sacrifices she endured."

Thao felt the emotion in this exchange and I could see that she was tearing up a bit.

"He's a good kid," she said. "I love him so much. He's really a good kid." Then mother and son hugged one another, very briefly.

The intensity in the room was overpowering. I felt it and had to restrain myself to not give Thao a hug as well.

I changed the subject. There was so much to disentangle about their family dynamics and about the psychological ramifications of Thao's insomnia.

"Ms. Tran, let me ask you. Does this restless condition always occur at night or do you also experience it in the morning?"

"First, it was at night, now it's also late afternoon when I work. I work as a nail technician in a nail salon. The job is really demanding and impossible. You know?"

"I bet. But are the symptoms worse at night?"

"Yes, they are worse. So much worse. I feel so restless. It's a burning sensation in my arms and legs, so I get up to move around. That helps."

"That's good to know. Does it get better when you massage your legs, or worse with caffeine?

"Doctor, it does. How do you know? Hot baths also help. I smoke sometimes and drink coffee. That makes it worse. I tried to quit smoking, but it has been so hard."

"Of course. Those two things certainly factor into it."

Vu added some interesting details.

"My mom's mood has been quite off lately. She has become depressed and is quite irritable. At most, I think she is getting about 5 hours of sleep per night and then she is off to the nail salon to work a 9-hour shift. She has become so withdrawn and vapid, as if she has no life left in her anymore. She was full of energy before, and now she has lost that zeal that encouraged me to do my best."

Thao was looking at her son askance, and although you could tell that she was not understanding everything her son said, she understood the gist of it. She turned her face to the side and down a bit, as if she was ashamed of what was happening to her.

Thao interjected here.

"Doctor, it's worse now during the holiday because I can't sit still. I may have to quit my job, but I have no money. Thank god Vu got his scholarship. Otherwise, I don't know what I'd do. I don't know how to do my job anymore with my legs feeling like this."

"Well, I think we can figure this out. Your symptoms are quite classic for restless legs syndrome, a condition where you don't have certain chemicals or neurotransmitters in the brain that control automatic movements. It's more complicated than that, and research is still being done in these areas. Occasionally, your iron storage may be low and you may have some damage to the nerves of the arms and legs, like from diabetes, so we have to check some labs. The underlying cause is unknown, but genetic influences play a strong role in the condition, particularly when the condition starts at a young age. The fact that this recently occurred makes me think that it's due to a secondary cause."

Thao's ears perked up a bit, as if she were both excited and scared.

I continued.

"The fact that you noticed this in the past 6 months is interesting. Have you recently had your blood checked for anemia? Any unusual menstrual bleeding lately?"

Vu interjected and relayed to me that his mother was recently diagnosed with fibroids and had had heavy menstrual bleeding. She had seen a gynecologist and they were waiting to see if she would need surgery. He hadn't thought about it but, yeah, he said, the two conditions appeared to have coincided.

Vu said, "What does that mean? Is there any significance between her being diagnosed with fibroids and the issue with her legs that prevents her from sleeping?"

"Yes, in this case, I think there is. Other than genetics, the two main reasons your mom may have developed this condition could be due to problems with her nerves, which does not seem to be the case here, and iron deficiency. Iron is needed to make a neurotransmitter in the brain called dopamine. Not having enough dopamine can cause a condition similar to what your mom is now experiencing."

"Wow. So, we can reverse her condition if we can figure out if she has iron deficiency anemia? Is that what you're saying?"

"Yes, potentially. I'll be ordering my own set of labs, such as a complete iron panel, complete metabolic panel, and labs to look for problems with the nerves. Restless legs syndrome, which I think your mom has, affects up to an estimated 20% of the population nationwide. The condition peaks in women ages 20 to 40 during their child-bearing years. In fact, one-third of pregnant women suffer from this condition, but the condition usually resolves after they give birth."

"With regard to my mom, do you think that once we prescribe her iron, her condition will improve? I can't see her going on like this. She is so tired from work. She then comes home and can't even sleep."

"That is the hope. But first we must check the blood levels of the different compounds that I mentioned. Then, depending on what her gynecologist says, she may have to remove her fibroids if they contribute to more bleeding. We must stop the source of the problem first. But, yes, potentially, if her iron is deficient, we can prescribe her that. Also, she should steer away from caffeine and nicotine, at least for the time being. Those things can worsen her RLS."

"What if it's not her iron? What do we do then?"

I could see the fire in Vu's eyes, a flame projecting vividly. He wanted to see his mom get better. He wanted her to sleep as if she hadn't slept before. She had sacrificed so much for him that it was now his turn to do the same. There was conviction there. There was so much caring from a family member, something that I hadn't seen for a long time in the sleep clinic.

"Well, there are a variety of medications, such as dopamine agonists or alpha delta 2 ligands, that she may respond to. However, let's first see what the labs reveal, and we can go from there."

"Sounds good, doctor. Thanks so much for explaining all of this. Mom, do you have any questions?

Thao was taking this all in. Her piercing, black eyes were fathomless. She smiled back, like she had understood all that her son and I had spoken about.

She asked, "What do I do in the meantime?"

"Well, as we discussed, avoid caffeine and nicotine. Soaking in a warm bath and massaging your legs can relax your muscles. Similarly, using heat or cold, and alternating between the two may lessen the sensations in your legs."

"Do I do this at day or night?"

"In the evening, before you plan to sleep. You would also want to establish good sleep hygiene because fatigue can worsen your symptoms. Of course, the RLS is not allowing you to sleep well, which increases your fatigue. But it's important that once your symptoms are a bit better, you establish good sleep hygiene. Also, getting moderate, regular exercise may relieve your symptoms, but try to do this during the day, not in the evening."

"But, doctor, I work during the day. I don't have time."

"I'm sure that you have a bit of a break at work. Use that opportunity to walk around and relieve some of that stress.

"Good idea."

"Yes, it is. Also, you may want to consider using a foot wrap that places pressure under your foot. This may also help. I want to see you back after you've had your lab work, so that we can address any issues that you may have and start you on therapy if we need to."

The mother and son thanked me. They appeared optimistic, armed with the new knowledge of Thao's condition. I saw them again, 2 weeks later, when Thao's lab results were available. As I had guessed, her iron level was low at around 20 ng per ml. We needed to increase that level to at least 50 ng/ml. No doubt—her fibroids were causing her anemia and she would need to have this surgically addressed.

In the interim, we decided that iron therapy (325 mg ferrous sulfate twice a day on an empty stomach) would alleviate her symptoms. I also instructed her that the iron should be given on an empty stomach an hour before eating or 2 hours after eating, along with 200 mg of vitamin C to increase absorption. We would then check her iron stores at 3 months to check the progress of her treatment. During this interim, she may also have undergone a myomectomy to remove her uterine fibroids, which would also give us a better idea of her progress. Last, I told Thao that if she couldn't tolerate iron or if her iron stores had not increased and her symptoms had not improved, an iron infusion—delivering iron directly into the blood—would be appropriate.

I didn't see Thao in 3 months' time as I requested, but her lab tests at that time were normal. Although she was lost to follow-up, I could only assume that her symptoms and sleep had improved. At least, I hoped so.

☾

Sleep Pearls

Let's look at some of the ways we can learn about and tackle RLS, as we did with Thao.

It's important to recognize that RLS is a clinical diagnosis and a sleep study or lab tests are not sufficient for a diagnosis. The key features of this condition can be summarized by the acronym URGE. The individual needs to experience the following:

1) An URGE to move the legs, usually associated with unpleasant leg sensations.
2) REST induces one's symptoms.
3) GETTING active, such as moving, walking, or stretching, offers relief.
4) EVENING or night worsens one's symptoms.

RLS can also be quite common during pregnancy; studies have shown that a quarter of pregnant women have this condition. A deficiency of folic acid or iron during pregnancy may trigger the condition. Also, there is some evidence that rising estrogen levels during pregnancy may contribute to it.

As with the other medical diagnoses we reviewed, such as Allen's sleep-disordered breathing, we need to be mindful that RLS is an imitator of insomnia. Also, patients with a hereditary form of RLS may experience an earlier onset of symptoms.

Certain deficiencies and medications or substances can also make RLS worse, such as various anti-depressants, iron deficiency, caffeine, nicotine, and alcohol. When you're experiencing insomnia, be aware of these restless behaviors that are causing it.

If the cause of the RLS is medication or deficiency of substances, then treatment of that condition or tapering off the medication usually resolves the problem. In those instances where the RLS is hereditary, without a predisposing condition, a variety of medications can be used, such as dopaminergic agents and medications for neuropathy, such as gabapentin.

It is important to realize that cognitive behavioral therapy for insomnia (CBT-I) is a guide and, although most will benefit from sequential sessions, as presented here, others will need to implement certain aspects of one treatment more than other aspects. However—and this is key here—you should not be introducing concepts that you may have learned in the past and are now including with CBT-I, whatever those may be. Although you can tailor the methods introduced here, you should not be mixing them with other techniques. While the sessions are relatively fluid, they build on one another and are meant to be followed sequentially to provide the most optimal results. There is a reason that the most important concepts of CBT-I, namely sleep restriction and cognitive restructuring, are situated in the middle portion of the program, after the basic concepts of sleep are explored. That said, you should follow the sessions in order, but you can spend as much or as little time learning the specific concepts as you wish. And while this program is intended to be 6 weeks in length, it can be prolonged or slightly shortened to meet your needs.

PART II

COGNITIVE BEHAVIORAL THERAPY FOR INSOMNIA (CBT-I)

Session 1

Understand Your Sleep

T O IMPROVE ONE'S SLEEP, ONE NEEDS TO UNDER-stand its basics. We need the alphabet of sleep to make sense of sleep. Cognitive behavioral therapy in insomnia (CBT-I), which is considered the cornerstone of long-term treatment for insomnia, is not as effective if we just know the lay of the land. We need to look for those crevices, a precise geography, to find where sleep lurks.

What is sleep and what is its purpose? Why do we sleep and why do we need it? At its basic level, sleep is what makes us feel good, what allows us to function optimally during the day. We just need it, like food for hunger and water for thirst. At a deeper level, though, sleep sustains life, conserves energy, repairs tissue, and is involved in consolidation of memory. The latter function has garnered a lot of press recently, as research suggests that suboptimal sleep may result in cognitive decline and memory impairment, as with Alzheimer's disease. Obviously, other factors such as genetics and the environment are involved in memory impairment, but we now know that sleep plays an essential role in this, as well.

But let's take sleep and dissect it, philosophically and literally. To put it simply, sleep is a state where awareness to stimuli is reduced and voluntary bodily functions are suspended. In comparison to a coma, which is a state of deep unconsciousness that lasts for an indefinite period as a result of a severe injury or illness, sleep is a reversible loss of consciousness characterized by diminished responsiveness that acts more or less predictably through stages. And what are those stages? Using a polysomnogram, or a sleep study, we can assess an individual's sleep through the electrical activity of the brain. The sleep study entails a variety of parameters like breathing and muscle movement, but, arguably, the electrical activity of the brain that can be determined via an electroencephalogram is the most important for our purposes here. The EEG allows us to determine the stages of sleep an individual undergoes throughout the night. During a sleep study, the sleep architecture (sleep stages) can be represented visually in a hypnogram, which is a visual representation of those stages of sleep.

The Stages of Sleep

When you are awake in bed, your wakefulness is characterized by high frequency (speed) and low amplitude (height) waves associated with body movements and eye blinks. We are fully conscious at this point, but, as we slowly drift to sleep, we enter the lightest stage of sleep, called Stage 1, or N1. It is at this point where there is diminished muscle activity and a slowing of our brain waves to theta waves, which occur at a rate of 5 to 8 times per second (noted in Hz). This is in contrast to the awake and relaxed activity of the brain—the alpha wave—which measures between 8 to 12 Hz. Stage 1 of sleep is considered so light that sleepers, and especially insomniacs, do not feel that they have actually slept when awakened during this period. The normal length of this stage is anywhere from 1 to 5 minutes and accounts for 2% to 5% of total sleep time.

During this quick introduction to sleep, the body enters Stage 2, or N2, which is the most common stage of sleep, representing 45% to 55% of total sleep time. Each cycle of this stage lasts about 10 to 60 minutes. In this stage and on an EEG, one can observe sleep spindles and K complexes, bursts of neural activity that are generated in the depths of the brain, in the thalamus. They signify that one has entered Stage 2 of sleep. It is now becoming progressively more difficult to awaken a person from sleep.

Perhaps the most interesting stage of sleep (besides REM sleep), is

Stage 3, or N3. It is also referred to as slow-wave sleep (SWS), which is important for memory consolidation. This stage is characterized by high amplitude and slow-wave activity, Delta waves occur in this stage, which occur at 1 to 4 Hz. Stage 3 constitutes about 10% to 20% of total sleep time, which accounts for 20 to 40 minutes during a typical sleep cycle. This stage is fascinating for many reasons. Many forms of parasomnias—abnormal behaviors while asleep—occur here. Sleepwalking (somnambulism), sleep talking (somniloquy), night terrors (pavor nocturnus), confusional arousals, and sleep-related eating disorder (SRED), among others. All find their homes here in this strangely exciting land.

And last, the belle of the ball, for better or worse, is Rapid Eye Movement, or REM sleep. This stage represents 20 to 25% of total sleep time and occurs in 4 to 5 episodes throughout the night. REM sleep is thought to be essential to memory consolidation and cognitive functioning. Dreams can occur in any stage of sleep, but they tend to be the most vivid, intense, and creative in this stage. I'm not being facetious when I call REM sleep the belle. Because most dreaming occurs in this stage (primarily fantastical dreaming), REM sleep has garnered the most attention due to its depiction in books and films on lucid dreaming. Films like Christopher Nolan's *Inception,* where a professional thief steals information by infiltrating the subconscious, has popularized lucid dreaming, where one can steer a dream in a direction that suits their purpose. REM behavior disorder (RBD) is a parasomnia that occurs in this stage of sleep where, because of dysfunction in the midbrain and pons, muscle activity is freed from inhibition and all sorts of havoc can occur.

These various stages of sleep are generally divided into Non-REM (Stages 1, 2 and 3) and REM sleep. The former stages occur during 75% to 80% of your sleep, while the latter comprises the rest. Slow-wave sleep, then, dominates in the first part of the night, while REM sleep becomes progressively lengthened and occurs in the last third of the night. It is no coincidence, then, that we tend to awaken having remembered a dream, although that dream dissipates quite quickly.

Just because one cannot remember a dream doesn't mean that they have not entered REM sleep. Contrary to popular thought, REM sleep can still occur in this situation.

How Much Sleep Is Necessary?

Now that we have discussed the specific stages of sleep, we need to understand how they change with aging because, after all, the amount of sleep one needs changes with age; if we adhere to the principle that everyone needs the same amount of sleep, one's perception of insomnia can become skewed. Newborns require up to 18 hours of sleep, which are broken into multiple short periods every 24 hours, with an equal percentage of active REM sleep and quiet NREM sleep. By 6 months, babies' sleep is significantly decreased to about 13 hours of sleep, over larger blocks of time. At 1 year of age, a baby's sleep pattern approximates a more adult pattern, where they sleep for longer periods at night and shorter ones during the day. During this time, they experience short REM periods immediately after falling asleep. But at 5 years of age, the child's sleep architecture begins to mirror an adult's, as those REM periods lengthen. Naps are, for the most part, abolished and the amount of sleep approaches an adult's sleep by 18 years of age.

As we reach adulthood, the amount of slow-wave sleep we need decreases. The reason for such a change could be because growth hormone is secreted in slow-wave sleep, and as we age, this hormone is not as essential anymore. REM sleep, however, remains relatively stable. In those who don't suffer from insomnia, the amount of time it takes to fall asleep, or sleep onset, is relatively stable throughout adulthood. But in general, the amount of time that is spent awake in the middle of the night, or wakefulness after sleep onset, increases with age. There are numerous reasons for this, such as getting up several times to urinate at night (nocturia), anxiety, and discomfort from chronic illnesses. The important thing to remember, and what most insomniacs don't realize, is that these awakenings are quite normal and don't become an issue unless one is unable to return to sleep once awake. This brings us to the question that sleep physicians are asked the most: Doctor, how much sleep do I need?

Again, just like sleep staging that varies with aging, the amount of sleep that one needs progressively decreases as we age, as previously mentioned. Focusing on adults, the average amount of sleep for optimal functioning is approximately 8 hours, with a range of 7 to 9 hours. Again, these numbers are averages, and one shouldn't adhere to obtaining the "perfect" number, because that number varies for everyone. In fact, one recent peer-reviewed study published in 2021 found that the cognitive scores of older adults who slept between 4.5 and 6.5 hours remained stable, which it termed the "sweet spot" of sleep. This doesn't mean that you should sleep in this range, but it does provide a glimpse into how our perceptions of ideal sleep are somewhat skewed.

Short sleepers, who comprise about 2% of the population, function optimally with approximately 6 hours of sleep, while long sleepers need at least 10 hours of sleep to feel alert. What most insomniacs hope to achieve is an "ideal" amount of sleep that forever seems out of reach. As we'll discuss later, when one begins to obsess about how much sleep one needs to obtain, it becomes problematic. Performance anxiety can set in. One is forever reaching for an ideal that one cannot attain. And in actuality, going to bed at 9 p.m. to ensure that one gets enough hours of sleep is counterproductive. It's best to retire to bed much later (assuming that one is unable to sleep at 9 p.m.) and spend more of your time in bed doing what it was meant for: sleeping, thus ensuring a better sleep efficiency. (We'll tackle this concept in Session 3.)

What Defines Insomnia?

So, what is insomnia exactly? It is defined as poor sleep quality characterized by difficulty falling asleep or staying asleep, awaking too early, and having nonrefreshing sleep. As readers may recognize, the consequences of insomnia include a lack of energy, fatigue, irritability, frustration, anger, and so forth. Acute insomnia, which affects 30% to 40% of adults during any given year, is defined as difficulty sleeping for between one night and a few weeks. On the other hand, chronic insomnia affects 10% to 15% of the US population, and is defined as difficulty sleeping for at least 3 nights per week for 3 months. To quantify and understand the gravity of the situation, more than 20 million people in the United States experience chronic insomnia. Insomnia increases with age and is more common in women, especially those who are postmenopausal.

Psychologist Arthur Spielman developed a model of insomnia that has proven useful to this day. It sets up certain factors that he describes as predisposing, precipitating, and perpetuating, which enable insomnia to develop and flourish. If insomnia cannot be related to psychophysiological or causal factors such as anxiety, depression, or pain, it is defined as primary insomnia, which usually develops in childhood and is more difficult to treat than regular insomnia. However, for the majority of insomniacs, who have secondary insomnia, or insomnia that develops later, their predisposition to developing insomnia is higher than those who don't experience insomnia. For insomniacs with a high predisposition, any precipitating event may set off the insomnia, as in our first case study of Laura, who first developed insomnia in the hospital while being treated for COVID-19, further perpetuated later by poor sleep behavior and cognition. It is indeed a vicious cycle whereby the original insomnia, which has now resolved, serves as a perpetuating factor to make itself viable again. It's as if the original insomnia has created a copy of itself to allow it to continue to replicate, like a virus. In Laura's story, for example, she was likely predisposed to insomnia because of her genetic makeup; her stay in the hospital simply precipitated that insomnia. Furthermore, because of her poor coping strategies and her cognitive arousal, she further perpetuated her insomnia.

Perpetuating factors for insomnia include a combination of cognitive arousal and conditioned responses to cues in the bedroom. Because CBT-I combats both of these issues head-on, it has remained a vital force in treating insomnia. Cognitive arousal includes excessive rumination at night, consequential fears of not obtaining good sleep to function adequately, and unrealistic expectations about sleep in general. Conditioned responses occur when certain cues in the bedroom are linked to insomnia, which induces a conditioned response to that alerting cue. (Laura's and Ava's stories, on pages 3 and 19, allow us to experience both of these perpetuating factors.)

Session 1 in Review:
What Can You Do?

Now that we have introduced the alphabet of sleep and the concepts underlying insomnia, it is time to tackle insomnia. The first assignment I usually like to give my patients after we go through the ABCs of sleep is creating a sleep log or diary, just as Laura does in Case 1 on page 3. This log should be completed when you awaken in the morning and it should be a rudimentary depiction of your current sleep pattern. There is no need to be precise here; this can actually be counterproductive. (We'll discuss this more on page 111.) Merely document when you go to bed, how long it takes you to fall asleep, if you awaken at night, and when you rise in the morning. Also, establish your goals for this program. For example, what is your ideal time for going to bed and waking? What is your purpose for undergoing such a program? Why now? Are you taking any sleep medications, and is your goal to discontinue them? Are there any environmental disturbances or medical conditions affecting your sleep? Again, the goal is to create a rough sketch of your sleep and what might be disrupting it so that we can know what to target. The more information that we have, the better we will become at honing in on the problem.

Session 2

Practice Sleep Restriction*

I N THE LAST SESSION, WE DISCUSSED VARIOUS ASPECTS of sleep, so that you could understand what we're tackling here. You should have had an opportunity to create your daily log for the week and to view a pattern of your sleep. You may have noticed that you wake up at a similar time every day, that you struggled to fall asleep, or that you fell asleep too quickly. You should've also noted whether you used sleeping pills to fall asleep, or if you exercised or obtained any sunlight in the morning when you woke up. We'll discuss all of these things, and more, in the ensuing sessions.

Good or bad, these facts you've taken note of are all insightful cues that you can use to your advantage. After all, if we don't know the precipitant or perpetuating factor of our insomnia, we cannot hope to solve it. And as you've likely gleaned by now, to improve your sleep, you must have a good understanding of your sleep: what works for you and what doesn't.

One of the most important topics in this session is the regulation of sleep as it applies to insomnia. Regulating your sleep involves mini-

---

* Note to readers: Anyone who is sleeping less than 6 hours a night and who has been diagnosed with epilepsy or bipolar disorder, is at high risk for falls, or has parasomnias should not try the sleep restriction exercises described in this session.

mizing chemical and environmental stimulants, but it can also involve an awareness of your sleep schedule and patterns.

Understanding Sleep Regulation

There are two key processes to remember when discussing sleep regulation. One is Process S, which is the homeostatic drive to sleep. It is essentially the accumulation of adenosine, a chemical sleep signal that continues to build up in your brain the longer you are awake. You can think of it as a desire for food. The longer one abstains from eating, the more likely is the desire to eat. However, once we sleep, that desire dissipates and builds itself back up again when we have been recharged from sleep. The cycle begins anew.

Certain compounds counteract adenosine, such as caffeine, which allows us to function if we are sleepy. For some insomniacs, caffeine may not be advisable in any amount. Most insomniacs have already recognized this fact. For others, they should avoid caffeine at least 6 hours prior to bedtime, or possibly even at noon. Alcohol is another substance that augments the role of adenosine by allowing us to initiate a quicker onset of sleep. However, given alcohol's short half-life, or the time it takes to excrete it from our system, its effect quickly wanes, allowing for nighttime awakenings. While alcohol can shorten REM sleep, it can also cause REM to rebound in the second half of the night with especially vivid dreaming.

Juxtaposed against Process S is Process C, the circadian altering signal. (You can remember C for Circadian.) Process C represents the circadian rhythm of arousal and counteracts our homeostatic drive to sleep. In other words, it creates a sort of balance, so that we can keep on going despite the fact that our drive to sleep is becoming stronger. Process C is not influenced by sleep deprivation, which is a good thing, because otherwise we could be sleeping throughout the day. There is a natural dip in the alerting signal, between 1 and 3 p.m., when we become sleepier. Contrary to fact, this dip in alertness has nothing do to with the aftereffects of the consumption of food (or the post-pran-dial effect) but, rather, with this lull, which, as research has shown, may be a productive outlet for tackling creative tasks. This is also a great time to take a short 15-minute nap without affecting one's sleep that night.

As we work on developing an ideal sleep schedule, we can stay mindful of these processes and how our habits are hindering or help-ing them. We'll discuss Process C in more detail in Session 3, but for now, remember that your sleep pattern is driven by your desire to sleep and your circadian rhythm.

Maximizing Your Sleep Efficiency

Cognitive behavioral therapy (CBT-I) is considered the gold-standard treatment for insomnia. Unlike sleep medications, which we'll address later in this chapter, treatment of insomnia with CBT-I is not only more effective than drugs but has lasting effects. It is usually offered as a 6-week program, but this varies with the individual and can be shortened to as little as 4 weeks. The mainstays of CBT-I are sleep restriction and stimulus control. This is recounted in the narrative of Laura, the advertising executive who began to experience insomnia after contracting the coronavirus (page 3). In this chapter, we'll pri-marily discuss sleep restriction.

The problem many insomniacs suffer from, and the reason we need to focus on sleep restriction as a solution, is that they do not have proper sleep efficiency. Sleep efficiency is a marker of how much of your time in bed is spent sleeping. We want to make sure your sleep efficiency is high, so that when you go to bed, you're able to sleep as much as pos-sible during that period. The goal is to limit your hours in bed to only those hours when you sleep. It does not make sense to spend 8 hours in bed if you only spend 6 of those hours asleep. Those 2 hours spent awake in bed will not only fuel anxiety about and frustration with one's inability to sleep, but they will also worsen and perpetuate insomnia.

This week, the goal is to determine the number of hours you spend in bed and the number of hours you actually sleep during that time. The formula you should use is the average amount of time asleep/average amount of time in bed × 100%. For example, if you go to bed at 9 p.m., spend 2 hours lying awake, sleep until 5 a.m., and awaken to spend another hour in bed, you have spent a total of 9 hours in bed. But only 6 of those hours were spent sleeping. Therefore, your sleep efficiency (6 hours / 9 hours × 100%) is 66%. If you slept the entire time you were in bed, you would have a sleep efficiency of 100%. You should calculate this for each night and each given week. You don't have to be exact with the numbers. An approximation is good enough. Once you calculate your sleep efficiency, you can then determine what modifications you can make to ensure that your sleep efficiency is as high as possible.

Sleep Restriction

Now we turn to improvements in your sleep schedule, based on your sleep efficiency. Here, we'll start honing the concept of sleep restriction, so you will feel comfortable extending or diminishing your time in bed. We often want a quick fix to insomnia, but this will take weeks, not days. Sleep restriction is one of the main tenets of CBT-I. No one likes to hear about decreasing time in bed, but as we discussed in our last week's session, over time, this can actually be beneficial. It is important to know that the majority of those with moderate to severe insomnia may have felt quite sleepy or fatigued during the previous week. As I mentioned previously, this is normal and should not discourage you in the least.

How do you know if and how you should sleep restrict? We have to look at your sleep efficiency. If your sleep efficiency is above 85%, you have the option of extending your time in bed by 15 minutes. You can either sleep-in later by 15 minutes or go to bed 15 minutes earlier. The choice is yours! You deserve it. If, on the other hand, your sleep efficiency is less than 80%, you will have to decrease your time in bed by 15 minutes by going to bed 15 minutes later. Remember that your wake-up time should always remain the same, no matter when you go to bed. You will maintain your sleep schedule from the previous week if your sleep efficiency hovers between 80 to 85%. You will neither be penalized nor rewarded. It is okay if you don't achieve a sleep efficiency of 85% right away. This may take some time, and you must understand that. A sleep efficiency of less than 80% is all right, too. You might become anxious about achieving a perfect 100%, but in Session 4, we'll discuss ways to prevent performance anxiety.

So, assess your sleep efficiency and then identify your time in bed by selecting a time period during which you actually sleep. For example, if you only sleep for 7 hours and need to awaken at 7 a.m. to get ready for work, then opt to go to sleep at midnight. If you're unable to fall asleep within 20 minutes, leave your bedroom and go to the living room to do something relaxing until you feel sleepy. The important thing is to never look at your alarm clock until it alerts you to wake up. Just approximate the time spent awake or asleep. (Many individuals can intuitively determine the time without looking at a clock, or at least estimate it.) If you happen to awaken earlier in the morning than your alarm and you cannot return to sleep, then you may want to start your day then. It is far better to awaken earlier and allow your homeostatic drive to increase than to linger and wallow in bed, hoping to catch minutes of sleep. Regular sleep patterns will strengthen your natural circadian rhythm and help you become grounded.

To be sure, and for the most of you, you will ultimately get less sleep than when you first began implementing CBT-I. This is normal and should not discourage you. In fact, this is an indication that you are progressing as you should. If you didn't feel tired, then it would mean your insomnia was probably not as bad as you imagined. Remember, the key to good sleep is adhering to a strict routine that fits your lifestyle. No two schedules will be the same, and it is up to you to determine how to approach it.

Anchoring your wake-up time is vitally important to sleep restriction. You must remember to awaken at the same time each morning (with the exception of the weekends, when you could allow yourself a 15- to 30-minute cushion) and get out of bed. Don't change this wake-up time. Only the time that you go to bed will be altered with a poor or robust sleep efficiency. Your wake-up time should remain constant.

Previously, you may have retired to bed at 10 p.m. in order to get more hours of sleep. But now you know better! If you're only obtaining 7 hours of sleep anyway, there is actually harm in going to bed earlier. For one, you will condition the bedroom environment as a place of torture, which will further perpetuate your insomnia. Furthermore, the inability to sleep for those 2 hours will fuel more anxiety and disrupt your sleep. Insomniacs would like any and every opportunity to be in bed longer, but, as I mentioned, this is counterproductive. Over the next few weeks, you may actually sleep less, but, over time, your homeostatic drive to sleep will get stronger and you'll sleep faster. More importantly, because of stimulus control, you won't be associating your bed with an inability to sleep.

Lingering in bed to allow yourself that transition is dangerous, precisely because we are weakening the link between the bed and sleep. Don't be tempted to just lie there and weaken the association that you have worked so hard to establish. Get out of bed and head to the shower or get ready for the day.

Have something to look forward to when waking up in the morning, even if this is just getting coffee at your local shop. As we'll discuss in the next session, you should make a point to obtain natural sunlight (or light from a lightbox) for at least 30 minutes. Establish an exercise regimen, either at the gym or outside. If you have a hobby or activity that you've fostered, make sure that you get up to create and enjoy those things. Establish accountability by arranging a meeting with a friend you do not want to disappoint. All of these examples will ensure you have a reason to get out of bed and start your day, however sleepy or fatigued you may be.

It is important to note your degree of sleepiness during the day while also remaining cognizant of the times when you are most alert. Most people feel sleepy in mid-afternoon while getting an evening surge of energy. We can take note of this, but you should not allow yourself to sleep or nap when you feel this way. The problem with naps is that it takes at least as long for people to fall asleep as it does for them to nap. As a result, such naps tend to be significantly longer than intended. Also, think back to our first session on sleep stages and how long they typically last. You will end up feeling much groggier when you awaken from a nap (especially if you wake up during REM sleep), and, although you may feel more energetic a few hours after, this will have diminished your sleep drive for the night. So, in short, unless the nap is absolutely necessary to perform an essential task, such as driving a long distance or going to work, then you should probably forgo a nap. As we'll discover in Bruce's case on page 79, shift workers can implement strategic naps. But on the whole, sleeping at every opportunity is not as good as it might sound. The goal is to sleep restrict so that the homeostatic drive, the Process S we discussed, will do its job and put you naturally to sleep (with the help of adenosine).

As you practice sleep restriction, take note of whether your sleep efficiency improves, or if you have setbacks. In these cases, it is important to consider other diagnoses that may be preventing you from gaining momentum, such as depression, sleep-disordered breathing, RLS, and so forth. An explanation of these diagnoses can be found on page 146. Others may find that they need to focus on aspects of CBT-I (like mindfulness, relaxation, and imagery) before they return and implement sleep restriction. We'll discuss this more in the following chapter.

Sleep Efficiency and Medication

At this point, we should probably discuss the role of sleeping pills and their implications for insomnia. One of the tenets of CBT-I is that it is a drug-free program, and that after 6 weeks, you should feel comfortable letting go of any pills you may be taking. This is easier said than done, because most of you have been taking hypnotics for some time and are ready to relinquish this. Although most practitioners would like the insomniac to discontinue their sleep medications prior to beginning the sessions, this can prove dangerous due to withdrawal effects of some of the agents, which we'll discuss below. It's more realistic to work alongside sleeping medications, weaning you off them while implementing CBT-I. Depending on the sleep agent, this may have to be done more cautiously, as with benzodiazepines, or more easily, with the use of over-the-counter agents such as diphenhydramine. Let's jump into the various classes of sleep agents.

In general, sleeping pills work by either blocking receptors of wakefulness or adhering to receptors that induce sleepiness. Sleep is promoted by chemicals such as adenosine, GABA, melatonin, and various cytokines. As you may recall, adenosine is a compound whose quantity increases the longer one is awake, and its buildup will result in sleep at a certain threshold. Once it has dissipated, the cycle starts anew until that threshold is reached again. Wake-promoting chemicals include histamine, hypocretin, serotonin, acetylcholine, and dopamine. As a result, sleeping pills that block such receptors induce sleepiness.

For the naïve insomniac, meaning that they haven't tried any sleeping pills yet, over-the-counter (OTC) agents are accessible and the first to be tried. One such example is diphenhydramine, an antihistamine, which is used in Benadryl and countless other PM agents. Although it may be useful for the few nights when one cannot sleep, this agent should not be a long-term go-to agent. For one thing, it can cause a hangover effect, which can be as bad as the effect of not having slept. Studies have found that chronic use of such agents can lead to cognitive impairment in older individuals. Another anti-histamine that has the same side effects as diphenhydramine, with more likelihood of dependence, is doxylamine. Antihistamines can cause sedation, dry mouth and throat, blurred vision, urinary retention, and constipation.

Although they may induce sleep, they are counterbalanced by their unpleasant side effects.

Melatonin is probably another popular OTC agent that is now being used not for its intended circadian effects but for its soporific (sleep-promoting) effects. Because it is a compound that the brain naturally produces, it is touted as being natural and effective. However, it can cause nightmares, headaches, dizziness, drowsiness, and daytime sleepiness. The effects vary with each individual, but the point is that even this purportedly innocuous compound can potentially have unwanted side effects.*

Another popular agent is marijuana, which exerts its effect via cannabinoid receptors. One form of cannabinoid is CBD, which has become quite popular for use for insomnia. Though CBD is considered generally safe, a study conducted in mice raised concerns about the potential for liver damage.† Other side effects of this agent include fatigue, diarrhea, and changes in appetite and weight.

Other OTC agents, which are not as popular as the above, include L-Tryptophan, valerian root, chamomile, and kava-kava. These agents have not proved to be useful for insomnia, although they are still touted for their sleep-promoting effects.‡ In the case of kava-kava, its safety concerns have included cases of hepatotoxicity, which has led to liver failure.§ It is important to understand that, depending on the study, the worldwide prevalence of insomnia is in 10% to 30% of the population. Given this enormous cohort of insomniacs and the potential revenue for treatment, it should not be difficult to understand

---

* Andersen, Lars Peter Holst, Ismail Gögenur, Jacob Rosenberg, and Russel J. Reiter. "The Safety of Melatonin in Humans." *Clinical Drug Investigation* 36, no. 3 (March 2016): 169–75.

† Huestis, Marilyn A., Renata Solimini, Simona Pichini, Roberta Pacifici, Jeremy Carlier, and Franceso Paolo Busardò. "Cannabidiol Adverse Effects and Toxicity." *Current Neuropharmacology* 17, no. 10 (October 2019): 974–89.

‡ Ibid.

§ Teschke, Rolf. "Kava hepatotoxicity: A clinical review." *Annals of Hepatology* 9, no. 2 (July–September 2010): 251–65.

why the pharmaceutical industry or even the OTC sleep aid market is so bent on improving sleep, even with compounds that have not shown any significant benefits in improving insomnia.* Just to place things in perspective, the revenue for OTC sleeping aids increased from $217 million to $429 million from 2011 to 2020. Not unlike big pharma, the OTC sleep aid market is continually (and silently) expanding while touting its natural composition and benign side effect profile.

On the other hand, we have the very conspicuous prescribed sleep agents that have been marketed so well over the past decade, agents such as Ambien, Lunesta, and Belsomra, which have become almost household names and a stand-in for sleeping pills in general.

In the beginning, barbiturates, originally used to treat seizures, were practically the only drugs used as sedatives and hypnotics between the 1920s and mid-1950s. However, due to their potential for overdose and withdrawal effects, they are no longer used to treat insomnia.

Benzodiazepines have largely taken over the space left vacant by barbiturates. They enhance the effects of GABA, the chemical that reduces the excitability of neurons. Untoward side effects of these agents include lethargy, delirium, risk of falls, long-term memory loss, and chemical dependence. If these medications are being prescribed for a long period of time, they need to be carefully weaned from the patient, as withdrawal effects can include a worsening of insomnia and seizures. Drugs in the category include lorazepam (Ativan), diazepam (Valium), alprazolam (Xanax), estazolam (ProSom), and so forth. As can be seen, the generic forms of these medications end with -pam or -lam, which makes for easy identification.

Antidepressants and antipsychotics agents make up another class whose agents sometimes also function as sleep aids. For example,

---

* Solomon, Daniel H., Kristine Ruppert, Laurel A. Habel, Joel S. Finkelstein, Pam Lian, Hadine Joffe, and Howard M. Kravitz. "Prescription medications for sleep disturbances among midlife women during 2 years of follow-up: a SWAN retrospective cohort study." *BMJ Open* 11, no. 5 (2021).

trazodone is heavily used by primary care physicians as a sleep aid at a lower dose than that used for its antidepressive effects. Its most significant, but rare, side effect includes priapism, which is a painful, persisting penile erection. Other effects include dizziness, hypotension, or lowering of the blood pressure, and abnormal heart rhythms. Silenor (doxepin) has also been used for insomnia and appears to have made a resurgence. Quetiapine (Seroquel), an antipsychotic, is also used for insomnia in the elderly who present with delirium. The important point about all these agents is that although they may modestly improve sleep, they present with numerous detrimental side effects that are quite worrisome. The side effects themselves include insomnia!

The stars of the show, however, have been and continue to be the benzodiazepine receptor agonists. You can blame this on the heavy marketing of these agents in the early 2000s or their popularization in the media, but, for good or bad, they have become the most recognizable sleep agents in the world. Drugs such as Ambien, Ambien CR, Lunesta, Intermezzo, and Sonata (less so) make up this class of hypnotics, which act on GABA to increase its receptors. This class carries the most memorable side effects, such as non-REM parasomnias (unusual motor activity) like sleepwalking, sleep-eating, sleep-driving, and so forth. Falls and memory impairment are also very common with these agents. Thus, although many insomniacs take these medications for a prolonged period, it is not advised.

The new kids on the block are the dual orexin receptor antagonists, medications like suvorexant (Belsomra), Lemborexant (Dayvigo), and daridorexant (Quviviq), which simulate the side effects of narcolepsy. (In narcolepsy, the amount of orexin is substantially reduced.) Because orexin antagonists resemble features of narcolepsy, their side effects also mirror the disease, which include sleep paralysis, hallucinations, and cataplexy-like symptoms. More common side effects include somnolence, headache, and dizziness. It is understandable that given these features, individuals with insomnia may be reluctant to take these types of hypnotics.

The question, then, is the efficacy of these agents. Given their preponderance and popularity, you may think that they have significant results, right? In general, these sleeping pills reduce the time to fall asleep by 10 minutes while they reduced the amount of time awake by, at most, 30 minutes. Moreover, the use of these agents beyond 2 weeks is discouraged, as they could cause falls (especially in the elderly), tolerance (higher doses are needed to exert the same initial effect), chemical and psychological dependence (becoming reliant and addicted to the medication), and rebound insomnia (a worsening of insomnia as one tries to wean off the agent).

Given these concerns and their limited efficacy, hypnotics are not the first choice of physicians, especially for chronic insomnias. They may offer a quick fix, and patients may ask for them, but this does not make them appropriate for everyone. Again, it should be only used for those with transient insomnia for a maximum of 2 weeks. The tools you have in hand now, derived from CBT-I, offer not only better results but also long-term efficacy.

Session 2 in Review:
What Can You Do?

Now that we have learned some essential tenets of CBT-I, let's delve into one of the first tasks at hand. Review your sleep log from last week. Determine the average hours you slept and your sleep efficiency for that week. (Again, sleep efficiency is the number of hours slept divided by the number of hours in bed).

Establish a consistent wake-up time to anchor your sleep and base the time you go to bed off of how many hours you typically spend sleeping. If you wake up, make sure to pull yourself out of temptation and remove yourself from the bed to avoid associating it with negative experiences. When you awaken in the morning, motivate yourself to get out of bed.

You should also evaluate whether any medications you're taking are conflicting with your sleep restriction practices. Continue to maintain your sleep log and calculate a sleep efficiency before the start of next week's session so you can adjust accordingly. Also continue to note any outside and environmental factors that may be disrupting your rest.

You may not have control over when you go to sleep, but you can determine when you wake up.

Session 3

Restrict Stimuli

A S WE CONTINUE THROUGH THE CBT-I SESSIONS here, we'll keep referring back to your sleep diary. In the last session we discussed finding your ideal sleep pattern and maximizing your sleep efficiency. But in this session, we want to pay attention specifically to the things that may have disrupted that efficiency. You may notice in your sleep journal that your sleep was affected by the environment, things that you experienced during the day, or any caffeine or alcohol you may have drunk. Inversely, you may have noticed that certain things may have improved your sleep, such as taking a warm bath prior to sleeping, resolving an argument you had or a dilemma you faced, or your inability to have slept well the night before. Now that we've started on the path of finding an appropriate sleep schedule, and rebuilding your drive to sleep via sleep restriction, we can start eliminating things that may be getting in the way of progress.

Circadian Rhythm and Light

Just as we discussed in Session 2, we have to be mindful of Processes S and C, and how we can support them. Sleep Process C is particularly sensitive to certain stimuli; it is specifically dependent on light and melatonin (particularly light). These are the signals that allow Process C to do its job. Light and melatonin are what we call zeitgebers, or "time givers" in German. They send signals to your hypothalamus, a portion of your brain responsible for letting it know when it's time to sleep. You can think of it as an alarm clock that resets every morning.

The process is as follows: light travels through our eyes and onto a pathway that terminates in the hypothalamus at a point called the suprachiasmatic nucleus. When light reaches this point, known as the central pacemaker, your brain essentially resets itself to "daylight," and begins "the morning." This is the reason why light at night, blue or otherwise, is especially problematic when initiating sleep. The brain cannot discern the difference between that light and daylight, and it will assume that it's morning. As such, light should be minimized at least 2 hours before sleep and, if it is absolutely essential for you to be in front of light for work functioning, a night mode can be activated on electronic devices to diminish light.

We can also use this same logic to bolster sleep by using light in the morning. Natural light, especially, or light from a light box, will train the brain to think it's morning, which it is. Insomniacs can experience poor sleep because they have lost the ability to receive light signals in the hypothalamus, so it is recommended that when an insomniac awakens in the morning, that they obtain at least 30 minutes of light, whether natural (best) or artificial (not as optimal), without the use of sunglasses so as to allow the light to enter their eyes and reach the hypothalamus. The timing of the light gets a little murky, but I will discuss this below.

Circadian disorders such as delayed sleep phase syndrome (DSPS) and advanced sleep phase syndrome (ASPS) often mimic insomnia. Savannah's story highlights this sleep disorder in Case 4 on page 39. The syndrome typically arises in adolescence but continues into adulthood if left unaddressed. Individuals with this sleep pattern have difficulty sleeping before midnight and, as a result, have difficulty rising in the morning. It is as if their rhythm has been skewed to the right, always a little delayed, and the objective is to advance it so that sleep occurs at a reasonable hour, mimicking the average person's. Of course, this disorder is not necessarily a disorder if the individual functions well and is able to sleep and wake up at a time that works for them. The problem arises when their circadian rhythm has to "match" or conform to others' schedules. Individuals with DSPS are often creative and do their best work at night. Treatment includes light therapy and melatonin. However, the timing of both of these options is crucial, because offering light earlier than needed will actually delay an individual's sleep further. Moreover, the dose and timing of melatonin should also be accurate. The dose for these individuals is significantly lower, usually 0.5 mg, and it should be taken at least 7 hours prior to sleep, instead of 30 minutes, as it is for the treatment of insomnia. Savannah's story discusses this treatment at length.

At the other extreme, we encounter ASPS, which may be less reported than DSPS because it tends not to exact the same societal pressures as DSPS. Individuals with ASPS tend to sleep early and wake early. They tend to be older, and they usually do not seek help for their problem, thinking this is just a part of aging. However, it is important to realize that this disorder can wreak as much havoc as the delayed form can. Mary's story on page 71 makes this abundantly clear, given that she cannot stay up with her husband and develops paranoia that her neighbor wants to steal her husband from her. What she cannot see at night, she attributes to secrecy and deception. This, of course, causes unnecessary anxiety and social pressures that could be avoided with the proper treatment, which would include light therapy and melatonin. However, the light is offered 1 hour prior to bedtime (unlike for DSPS, for which light is offered when the individual awakens) and melatonin is administered in the morning. The treatment is recounted in Mary's story.

Stimulus Control

Stimulus control is highly useful in treating insomnia and can be considered a partner to sleep restriction because it helps maximize sleep efficiency by limiting disturbances. Stimulus control is based on the concept of conditioning and association. Its goal is to reassociate the bed or bedroom with sleep, so as to alleviate the anxiety linked to sleep.

To this end, one must begin the process of only associating the bed with sleeping and relaxation. The bed must only be used for sleeping or sex. It is not a place where one works; pays the bills; or watches Netflix, Apple +, or the like. This may be difficult for those who live in a small living space where a room is multipurposed but, even in such a setting, the bed can be partitioned and set off from other work-related tasks. The goal is to create a strong link between the bed and sleep and to sever anything that diminishes such a connection between the two. The goal for you is to sleep when you see a bed. We must forge that strong link.

If you do everything in bed, then nothing is sacred in bed. And sleep is golden. So limit, or ideally do away with, any menial tasks that you've been doing in bed. The less you do in bed outside of sleep, the more you will come to associate your bed with sleep automatically, which can be extremely helpful to the brain when you're finally lying down at the end of a long day.

As you'll remember, you should also keep any sensory stimuli or environmental factors outside the bedroom. Minimize light, noise, or any other distraction from the outside. Sometimes this is impossible, like if a roommate is talking to someone too loudly while you're trying to sleep. Talk to them and explain that they're affecting your sleep. If they appreciate their own sleep, they'll understand. With regard to light, a recent study showed that individuals who slept with a television or light on were more likely to gain weight and develop obesity. Researchers determined that being exposed to light at night may affect levels of melatonin, leading to changes in circadian rhythms and weight gain from altered eating habits. Yet another recent study revealed that exposure to a moderate amount of light while sleeping with the eyes closed increased resistance and altered glucose metabolism. Furthermore, this exposure to light also increased sympathetic activity, as observed by an increased heart rate and elevation of cortisol.[*] All of this is to say that

---

[*] Phyllis C. Zee. "Proceedings of the National Academy of Sciences." March 14, 2022.

one's environment during sleep is especially important. Do all that you can to minimize it and bathe yourself in that cocoon state.

The idea of a buffer zone and relaxation time can also help you set boundaries about when you might start reducing stimuli and light. Both the buffer zone and scheduled relaxation time are intended to lull and transition you from the hectic schedule of the day to the peaceful slumber of night. As I've mentioned before, for most, sleep is not a light switch that you can turn off or on at a moment's notice. It is a gradual process, and so the techniques you use to prepare for sleep must be taken seriously. A buffer zone creates that transitional time before sleep when you can progressively unwind. No work-related activities or strenuous physical activities should be performed at this time. The idea is to relax. Listening to music, reading a book, or practicing yoga are activities that are conducive to such an idea. Music and reading can even extend to the bed, as long as the duration is short. Music should be relaxing and, ideally, soothing, conjuring pleasant images. Reading in bed should last no more than 15 minutes and should consist of novels that take you to a fictional domain and distract you from life stressors. However, stay away from tablets and stick to a traditional paper format, even if the tablet light is dim and doesn't emit blue light. Taking a warm bath is actually a great idea, too, not only because it relaxes the muscles but because the temperature gradient one experiences entering and leaving the tub cools the body significantly and leads to better sleep. A cool temperature is optimal for sleep, whereas a warm or hot one is not.

Some people tend to worry a lot when they go to bed. Often, an insomniac lies in bed and ruminates about the problems they have faced or, more often, will face in the future. The anxiety this fosters further contributes to insomnia. (Ava's narrative in Case 2 on page 19 is an example of an unruly and repetitive meditation that is counterproductive to sleep.) We want to avoid this; after all, it runs counter to this rest time that we're trying to establish before bed. A great way to combat worrying and preserve your established relaxation time is to create a designated time to worry. This may not sound so pleasant, but it is a great way to separate chaos from the peaceful promise of sleep.

You can schedule this time earlier in the day, perhaps after dinner. If the time of day is too early, however, you may have forgotten what you wrote down and may have a propensity to ruminate again once you retire to sleep. It is better to write these problems down on a piece of paper (and paper is better in this regard that an electronic tablet or phone because it does not use the blue light that is detrimental to sleep) and stop ruminating about them while going to sleep. You just need a receptacle for these thoughts that intrude into your sleep. Recognizing that they exist and compartmentalizing them is one way to simultaneously broach and address them to deter them from intruding into sleep. These thoughts need not be problematic, either. Some people simply worry about getting up in time to make lunch for work or decide what to wear the following day. The solution to these issues is fairly easy: Address these issues before you go to sleep. That is, fix the lunch and lay out your clothes, so you don't have to worry about it the following day. Preparation and routine are key to good sleep. The less that you have to worry about, the more restful your sleep will be.

Relaxation techniques, such as deep breathing exercises (particularly the 4-7-8 model, which we'll discuss in the next session), mindfulness, guided imagery, and others are also instrumental in combating insomnia. The idea is to distract your mind from sleep and focus on things over which you have control. Insomnia is fostered by a lack of control, and the idea is to regain control over that which one can potentially control. You may not have a choice about when you fall asleep, but you can control those ideas that can allow for a peaceful slumber. For example, using the technique of guided imagery, you can imagine an ideal situation in which you may have participated, such as a glorious vacation in Santorini, and allow that thought to pervade your consciousness. This not only allows you to think about something other than sleep, but it also predisposes you to positive thoughts that will allow you to relax. Each individual has their own way of relaxing, so the ideas above may not apply to everyone. But, in general, certain activities should be avoided before going to bed, such as work-related activities, finance, physical exercise, and family matters that may contribute to arguments.

Of course, some of this is unavoidable, such as when a big project at work is looming, but this allows for an opportunity to plan these tasks beforehand so as to not allow them to pervade into your buffer time. Remember: The more you address any issues that may be contributing to poor sleep before you go to bed, the more you have control over the situation, which, ironically, will allow you to relinquish control to sleep. You must have control in order to give up control and let go.

An Integrative Approach to Insomnia

An integrative approach to insomnia, which emphasizes the Noise Reduction Approach for Insomnia (NRAI), is also essential in the CBT-I arsenal. This concept, which has been reiterated by Rubin Naiman, PhD, refers to sleepiness as the inclination to sleep and noise to any stimulation that interferes with that sleep. Noise can emanate from the body, mind, and the bed.

Reduction of body noise can occur when one is attuned to the physiology of the body that could be interfering with sleep, whether this be addressing one's medical disorders, medication and substance use (such as caffeine and alcohol), or health concerns common to women, such as premenstrual or menopausal symptoms. The goal of a mind-noise reduction is to decrease hyperarousal, which CBT-I accomplishes rather well with the use of sleep hygiene, stimulus control therapy, sleep restriction therapy, and relaxation techniques.*

A reduction in bed noise is accomplished by maintaining a healthy sleep environment, which can mean using HEPA filtration systems, decreasing electromagnetic fields that can suppress natural melatonin levels, and using organic bedding that is free of pesticides. In addition, the bedroom should be treated as a sanctuary or a retreat from the waking world, so that all "outside" worries can be prevented from entering

---

* Rakel, David. "Insomnia." In *Integrative Medicine*, 74–85. Philadelphia, PA: Elsevier, 2017.

"within." Exposure to electronics and anything that is a reminder of waking, such as a clock or a phone, should be avoided. If one does not feel physically or psychologically safe in the bedroom, installing a security system or using religious material to establish a sense of safety is also essential. In short, an integrative model of healthy sleep emphasizes each of the domains that can diminish the noise of insomnia.

Session 3 in Review
What Can You Do?

If you're in a sunny climate, make sure you get at least 30 minutes of light (natural light is best but a sleep box with artificial light of at least 10,000 lux will also work). This will reset your circadian rhythm and allow your brain to think that you have started a day—a natural and more effective alarm clock!

Only use your bed for sleep—to make the connection between your sleep and the bedroom environment more robust. If you cannot fall asleep within 20 minutes of going to bed, leave your bedroom and head to the living room to browse through magazines or conduct dull activities with minimal light.

Noise, light, and other sensory stimuli run counter to sleep, and they should be minimized when attempting to sleep. Even a miniscule amount of light has been shown to be detrimental during sleep, with the potential to create health problems (diabetes mellitus, obesity, etc.). If light is a problem, make sure to invest in a good sleep mask that entirely covers the eyes.

Also, ensure that you create a buffer zone prior to going to bed, where you can transition naturally from activity to passivity. Sleep is a dimmer and not a light switch that can be turned on and off at a moment's notice. Recognize that you may need to engage in relaxing activities other than work, such as yoga, listening to music, reading, and deep breathing exercises, to allow this natural segue.

An integrative approach to sleep medicine also emphasizes noise reduction, whether this noise emanates from the body, mind, or the bed itself. Ensure that your bedding is optimal, that electronic equipment is avoided, and that you feel physically and psychologically safe in your sleep cocoon.

Session 4

Open Your Mind to Cognitive Restructuring

THIS WEEK MAY PERHAPS BE ONE OF THE MOST important in our immersive CBT-I program. The reason I say this is we will be primarily focusing on mood and irrational thoughts this week, both of which play an immense role in sleep. You may know this because our mood dictates how we feel when we sleep. If we are mad or excited when we go to sleep, we may sleep less that night. Hearing distressing news or arguing with others is not conducive to sleep. We have all experienced this. Similarly, when we are relaxed and know that we have things under control, our sleep is much smoother and insomnia may not rear its head at all, even for hard-core insomniacs.

As we've discussed, our environment also plays a significant role in our ability to sleep. A space that is too loud, too warm, too cold, or too well-lit will adversely affect our sleep. We sleep best in a cocoon-type setting, and any stimulus that throws this off balance will detrimentally affect our sleep. You may have experienced this if you were sleeping next to a house that was having a loud party, or have had family members or friends who were speaking or arguing loudly while you were trying to fall asleep. The noise itself is a factor in not allowing you to sleep—it is a repetition, or something that intrudes upon your calm atmosphere. However, what is probably more detrimental is the feeling that that noise engenders. You no doubt have felt anger toward the individual(s) causing that noise and harbored resentment toward them when they're having fun while you are sleeping in an environment that, in your mind, resembles hell. As an example, you can visit Izzie's and Allen's narrative, where Izzie felt such intense anger toward Allen for his abominable snoring. It is important that when you go to bed, you let that negative energy flow from you and instead focus on your sleep. It may also help to remember that most individuals do not recognize that their noise is affecting your sleep. They are not intentionally trying to prevent you from sleeping, but, at that moment, you have become too self-aware and everything becomes personal. You're thinking: Why should I be suffering from their stupid and selfish behavior? Why do they act the way they do when they know I need my sleep to function tomorrow? Again, they may not know the hurdles you're up against. Some individuals can sleep soundly even in a noisy environment, and so they may reason that this applies to you, too. If this situation persists, you may have to calmly address your inability to sleep and politely ask that they refrain from anything that may not be conducive to your sleep. Almost all will apologize for their careless behavior and will be mindful of your request. In those circumstances where this unwanted behavior persists, you may have to resort to more serious confrontation, but I've found that these instances are rare.

Similar to emotion, negative and irrational thoughts will also adversely affect your sleep. No doubt, once you are in bed, all sorts of thoughts will invade your mind, anything from the work that you have to complete tomorrow to financial issues that are a cause of concern. Because sleep is a solitary process, you also have a great deal of time (the entire night!) to think about your problems and work through all the scenarios that may arise by yourself. Not only is this a daunting task, but it becomes problematic because you have to confront these issues alone and in a state of irrationality, especially if you are sleep-deprived. As we previously discussed, writing such concerns and thoughts down before you sleep may alleviate the rumination you experience. Also, such writing helps to transfer what is in your mind onto paper, so that you can focus on it at a later time. If you think of yourself as a computer, you have just moved the thought from the hard drive (brain) into the soft drive (paper). Once you get the hang of this transference of negative energy, we can also start to examine additional mood-related sleep obstructions.

Catastrophizing and How to Avoid It

False beliefs about sleep or other subject matters adversely affect our sleep. We see this most prominently in Ava's case on page 19, but you might notice that it's a common thread between a lot of my patients. In a state of hyperarousal (as occurs with insomnia) or sleep deprivation, the mind ruminates about anything, whether this be logical or illogical (primarily the latter). The most common illogical thought that occurs as we experience insomnia is the effect it will have on us the subsequent day. We feel that we cannot function adequately at work or home and this will affect our performance, which would ultimately lead to disastrous consequences. You may convince yourself that you are close to termination at your job, or that your loved ones are annoyed with you, or that you will sustain a potentially hazardous car accident. . . . This is called catastrophizing, and we can counter this irrationality by recalling how few instances there are when our fears have actually come to fruition. Again, think back to Ava's irrational fears that never transpired!

If you experience insomnia most nights, and if you have convinced yourself that your insomnia is putting you in grave danger, the percentage of these occurrences must be high. In other words, if your insomnia was a legitimate cause of termination, or a breakup, or more, then you would be experiencing these things all the time. But reality tells us this is not so. You may want to actually formulate evidence for these occurrences to see that the evidence does not conform to reality and write these down. As always, writing is helpful because if these thoughts occur again, you have already dismissed them as not worthy of further elaboration. Evaluating your thoughts in light of this new evidence, you may want to modify your initial irrational thought and rephrase it in a way that is realistic. For example, if the irrational thought is that you will get fired if you don't sleep and perform your best (as occurred with Ava), rephrase it in a way that conforms to what actually happened in the past in your bouts with insomnia: "I may not perform my best at work and may be irritable, but I will get through this day without being terminated. With the new CBT-I techniques that I have learned, I will have better nights and better days at work. It will take some time, but it will happen!"

You should also think about everything else you have learned about sleep in general and debunk those myths. For example, recognize that you may not need 8 hours of sleep, a thought that could have guided your perception of perfect sleep and the inability to attain this holy grail. For example, a recent study conducted at Washington University School of Medicine showed that the "sweet spot" of sleep is actually 6.5 hours, where cognitive performance is stable over time. Also, recall that going to bed early may actually be detrimental because your inability to fall asleep at that time may make the connection between your bed and sleep less robust.

Instead, recognize that your best option in this situation is to prolong the time that you go to bed, so that you can not only build up a greater homeostatic drive to sleep but also to sever the links between your insomnia and the bed or bedroom environment. Looking specifically at the homeostatic drive to sleep, you may recognize that the nights you did not sleep well actually led to better nights subsequently. This is because the drive to sleep has had time to build up to naturally put you to sleep. (Recall the role of adenosine in this situation and how its buildup and dissipation are related to your sleep.)

The "Fuck It All" Approach

Although this approach doesn't exactly fall under the repertoire of CBT-I, it is one that I have found helpful with some patients over the years, especially for those who have difficulty rephrasing their worries. This approach essentially pushes the catastrophizing concept to such an extreme degree that when it comes to ruminating about the problem, one has already encountered the worst-case scenario and has grappled with it, at least in theory.

The issue with catastrophizing is that one is projecting into the future what they fear will occur if their insomnia persists. For example, we can again refer to Ava and her fear of getting fired. She catastrophized about the possible occurrence of this termination, although it never occurred. Her anxiety was about the future and the possibility of being fired. The "fuck it all" approach pushes the envelope to the most extreme degree so that one has already encountered this fear.

As we've just discussed, fear plays a big role in the perpetuation of insomnia—fear of the unknown, fear of what could happen, fear of being powerless to do anything about it. However, this modern approach allows one to directly confront the fear of not being able to sleep and approach it actively and realistically.

In the case of Ava, for example, such an approach suggests that Ava think that she has already been fired, her worst-case scenario of her inability to sleep. So, Ava has been fired, now what? Thinking logically, she has many options now that she has been terminated. She can apply for a new job, she can change careers, she can take that time to pursue her interests, and so forth. This approach suggests that we encounter that fear, look it in the eye, and then move on.

Meditating For Sleep

Next, we will tackle the role mindfulness plays in alleviating insomnia. Many of you may have had some experience with this. In short, mindfulness is a form of meditation in which one perceives things as they are occurring at the moment without judgment or interpretation. In other words, you concentrate on the "here and now" as opposed to the "there and future."

Mindfulness involves muscle relaxation, breathing methods, guided imagery, and other relevant techniques. For example, its main tenets

involve muscle relaxation and breathing exercises. It is also important to meditate and engage in mindfulness during the day to help
strengthen your brain and prime it for the night, when you're ready
to sleep.

With muscle relaxation, you'll focus on the different parts of your
body and how they relate to it as a whole. Tighten your muscles one at a
time, and then relax them. Tighten your abdominal muscles and then
relax them. Close your eyes forcefully and then open them. Curl your
toes and then straighten them. The goal is to focus on the present and
the control that you have over your body. It is control that can apply to
your other endeavors. Realize that you are in charge of your body, of
your sleep, of your life.

Similarly, breathing exercises help you to stay in the moment.
Before sleep (during your uninterrupted cushioned time before going
to bed) find a quiet environment, whether this be the bath or a small
space in your living room—but not the bedroom environment—and
practice deep breathing. Deeply, and slowly, breathe in and out. You
may also want to utilize the 4-7-8 breathing pattern, also known as
the relaxing breath, which involves breathing in for 4 seconds, holding
the breath for 7 seconds, and exhaling for 8 seconds. The breathing
pattern is based on pranayama, which is an aspect of yoga that per-
tains to the control of breathing. Not only does this technique help you
to diminish anxiety and control responses such as anger, but it also
decreases heart rate. Initially, only 4 breath cycles in a row should be
attempted, as this technique can cause lightheadedness. However, over
time, once an individual is acclimated to the technique, the results can
be overpowering. This breathing technique can not only be utilized
for insomnia but for other stressful situations, as well. Our relaxation
response is mediated by the vagus nerve, and one way to engage this
nerve is to conduct this deep breathing exercise. Dr. Andrew Weil, an
integrative medicine specialist at The University of Arizona, has even
called the relaxing breath a "natural tranquilizer for the nervous system"; it increases heart rate variability, which is a good thing. When
we inhale, our heart rate increases and, when we exhale, the heart

rate decreases. Heart rate variability is beneficial because the greater it is, the greater the efficacy of the heart to pump blood to our various organs and muscles.

Another relaxation technique that is highly useful and can serve as another tool in our armamentarium against insomnia is guided imagery. Guided imagery allows you to recreate a setting in which you may have felt your best, whether this be an event, a relaxing locale, or anywhere else, and imagine yourself there again. Alternatively, you can imagine a setting in which you have never been but have always imagined as a tranquil spot, your own private Shangri-la, whether this be an isolated island with no intrusion from anyone or anything, a favorite spot with your loved one(s), or up in space. It really doesn't matter, so long as it's personal to you. Think of it as a teleportation, one where you, alone, are in control of your destiny. In this scenario, you should immerse yourself in all the senses—visual, olfactory, aural, gustatory—and practice a sort of mindfulness. Imagine how you would interact with the flora and fauna in your imagined space, how you would act toward this environment, and how you would conduct yourself. Not only will the halcyon scene relax you, but it will introduce a distraction from your insomnia. Think back to Jeremy's story, where the town in which he felt the most relaxed and peace with himself was the imaginary space where he "teleported" himself when he couldn't sleep. When insomnia occurs, you should detach yourself from anything related to the bed or bedroom environment by either physically leaving it or mentally teleporting yourself elsewhere.

Another relaxation technique that some of my patients have found useful is to be lulled into sleep, like a baby. Meditative stories, either via podcasts or apps like HeadSpace, allow another avenue in which to feel relaxed and less anxious. The soothing and often soporific voices these narrators use are in direct contrast to the bustling noise of the workday. The result is a hypnotic trance that may allow you to sleep quicker. Heart rate and breathing will slow, which increases the chances of obtaining falling and staying asleep faster.

If you usually read in bed, don't be afraid to continue this habit. Light reading can help you quickly fall asleep, especially if it's fiction. Studies have shown that fiction allows you to escape the realities of the present day to a remote place, where you are implicated in someone's else predicament, not your own. Not only does this allow for empathy, but it also helps you forget about your problems. When the brain is occupied, the body's fatigue takes over and allows sleep to occur naturally. Reading until one is so tired that they cannot focus on the words is a good strategy.

Again, these techniques can be used not only for insomnia but for any situation in which you find yourself stressed. Remember: sleep is an extension of your life. What affects your daily, active life will also affect your slumber. Take this to heart and allow yourself to exercise some of these techniques we've learned that are also applicable to your day-to-day activities.

Session 4 in Review:
What Can You Do?

The most important lesson for this session is to try and stop catastrophizing when attempting to sleep. We are at our most irrational when we cannot sleep because we have ample solitary time to ponder everything, making life-and-death propositions that do not necessarily reflect reality. When this occurs, rationalize and determine whether any of these scenarios have occurred or will realistically occur in the future. Better yet, write your thoughts on paper an hour prior to sleep and focus on it later when your mind can better evaluate the situation.

Also, don't forget to engage in meditation, whether this be mindfulness, muscle relaxation, breathing exercises, or guided imagery. You'll find that these techniques will make you calm by activating the parasympathetic system, and more importantly, allow you to focus on something other than your inability to sleep. Reimagine sleep, and allow your senses to transport you to your own private and serene Shangri-la.

Session 5

Fine-Tune Your New Sleep Habits and Identify Hurdles

A S WE ENTER THE FINAL STAGES OF CBT-I, RECOGNIZE that you've learned some very powerful techniques—sleep restriction, stimulus control, and meditation and mindfulness—that have improved your sleep. These techniques will need to be honed, and not everyone will have the quick results they hoped for. This will take some time, and so one must be patient. However, for those who have stayed the course and have not made any headway, we must consider other causes for your insomnia, fatigue, and daytime sleepiness. This week, we will focus on some common medical conditions and sleep disorders that can either contribute to your insomnia or simulate insomnia.

First, recall the definition of insomnia we introduced in our first session together: difficulty initiating sleep, maintaining sleep, or awakening too early in the morning. Now, if you have tackled these difficulties and are still feeling fatigued or sleepy, then other medical causes or sleep disorders need to be entertained. It is important to differentiate between fatigue and sleepiness because the two do not equate. Fatigue is extreme tiredness, which does not necessarily result in sleepiness. In fact, with insomniacs, fatigue is often synonymous with the inability to sleep, which results in frustration and irritability. Imagine yourself hungry and not being able to eat. The same holds true for fatigue and the inability to sleep when you most need or desire it. On the other hand, sleepiness is the state of being sleepy and having the great like-lihood of falling asleep. That is the reason fatigue is so problematic for those with insomnia: at the moment you desire sleepiness, you're deprived of it.

Identifying Lifestyle Challenges to Sleep

When you consider the success you've had with your sleep but are still feeling fatigued or sleepy, think about other reasons for this, includ-ing your diet. We may not realize how important diet is to sleep, but research has shown that one's diet is vital to good sleep.

For example, high-carbohydrate meals with high glycemic indexes can affect energy levels and sleep, resulting in increased awakenings at night and diminished slow-wave sleep. Both of these do not portend well for good sleep quality. Both the Mediterranean diet (which incorporates plant-based and high-fiber foods, as well as lean meats) and the DASH diet (which focuses on avoiding foods with high salt and saturated fat and promotes food with high levels of fiber, potassium, and magne-sium) are examples of diets that work to not only keep you healthy but also promote quality sleep. Meanwhile, foods that are rich in melatonin, which can also help promote good sleep, include tart cherries, goji ber-ries, eggs, milk, fish, and nuts (especially pistachios and almonds).

In what turns out to be a vicious cycle, eating food that does not agree with the guidelines above could result in hormonal changes in your body that would adversely affect your sleep. For example, the produc-tion of the hormones leptin and ghrelin are thrown off balance in those who are sleep-deprived and makes it easier for them to gain weight.

Furthermore, gaining weight can cause other sleep disorders to rear their heads, a principal one being sleep-disordered breathing, such as obstructive sleep apnea. We'll discuss this later.

Lack of exercise can also derail quality sleep. Although researchers don't know the precise mechanism by which exercise improves sleep, we do know that moderate aerobic exercise increases the amount of slow-wave sleep while also stabilizing and decompressing your mood, which all lead to quality sleep. The timing of exercise has always been in contention, with some arguing that exercise should be limited to the morning or afternoon hours. However, exercising 2 hours before going to bed is also beneficial; the endorphins released with exercise have had time to be cleared, allowing for a wind-down period. Furthermore, although exercise elevates one's core body temperature, it is the steep decline of that fall after a couple of hours that helps to facilitate sleep. The exercise need not be long. You may notice a significant difference with just 30 minutes of moderate exercise, which does not necessarily need to be aerobic. Any exercise will increase your heart rate and elevate your temperature, so select one that fits your ideal needs, whether this be running, yoga, Pilates, power lifting, or spinning.

This is akin to taking a warm bath (not shower) at night, which also improves sleep. Researchers have found that bathing 1 to 2 hours (ideally, 90 minutes) before sleep can lead to a better quality of sleep with a faster onset. Because sleep occurs better in a cooler environment, a warm bath stimulates the body's thermoregulatory system, so that blood is diverted from the core body to the hands and feet. Moreover, once we bathe and leave the bathtub, that steep change in temperature allows the body to cool down further and faster. The drop in temperature also alerts the pineal gland in the brain to secrete melatonin and begin the transition to sleep. Ensure that you take the bath for an optimal time of 10 minutes.

Warm showers at night are not as conducive to sleep as baths (and they even be more detrimental), primarily because a shower has an alerting quality to it, signaling that it may be time to start the day. Also, unlike a warm bath, water from a shower doesn't surround the body and can't create that similar layer of insulation. Given the fact that the sleep is better in a cool environment, you may think that immersing your body in cold water before sleep can also be helpful. However, this strategy is actually counterproductive because not only is the cold water an alerting signal, but it can also initiate a fight-or-flight response, because the temperature drop is too erratic. The ideal temperature for good sleep is approximately 65°F, although a temperature of up to 72°F may be more ideal for those who prefer a bit more warmth. Because our core body temperature continues to decrease in the evening prior to sleep, a cool environment mirrors this drop and improves quality of sleep. Furthermore, a cooler environment promotes melatonin production, which also favors better sleep. However, it is important to realize that one's temperature preference is idiosyncratic, and some may sleep well even in a warm environment. However, even if one prefers the warmth, it may be a good idea to decrease the temperature just a bit to see if this improves your sleep. Experiment and see where this can lead you.

Identify Medical Challenges to Sleep

Other factors that can derail your sleep are medical conditions that contribute to or mimic insomnia. As we see in the case studies in this book, some patients who present with insomnia, such as Allen and Thao, may later be diagnosed with obstructive sleep apnea and restless legs syndrome, respectively. Often, insomnia is part of a parcel that coexists with other diagnoses, both medical and psychiatric. If you don't improve with the techniques that were presented in the first four sessions, then it's time to consider the diagnoses below.

Probably the most common medical condition and sleep disorder that mimics or causes insomnia is sleep-disordered breathing, of which obstructive sleep apnea is the most recognized. Obstructive sleep apnea occurs when the muscles that support the soft tissues in the throat temporarily relax and cause the airway to become constricted. As a result, breathing is momentarily halted or decreased, which results in diminished oxygen. Because of this diminished oxygen, one awakens to reinitiate breathing (called an arousal). Some of those with this condition can return to sleep, although they are usually fatigued and/or sleepy in the morning as a result of these awakenings. However, others awaken from this relaxation of the airway and diminished oxygen level and are unable to return to sleep. This results in sleep maintenance insomnia, whose cause the patient may not know.

All they recognize is that they awoke in the middle of the night and were unable to return to sleep. (Think back to Allen's narrative; he was brought to the clinic because both he and his wife were affected by his snoring.)

Obstructive sleep apnea is not innocuous. Studies have shown that, if untreated, this condition can cause hypertension, cardiovascular issues, irregular heart rate, depression, strokes, and heart attacks. So, basically, a lot. More recent studies have shown a correlation between obstructive sleep apnea and dementia, as with a lack of sleep. Although approximately 70% of patients with obstructive sleep apnea are obese, 30% have normal weight and body habitus. However, this latter group has facial features that predispose them to this condition, such as an elongated face and a small jaw. If you think of your mouth as a house, anything that can contribute to a small area may also increase your chances of a breathing disorder. Too often though, as Allen's case shows, these patients are dismissed as insomniacs without a need to investigate further. Because their body habitus is in the normal range and they don't fit the picture of someone with obstructive sleep apnea (i.e. overweight, large neck, medical issues, and so forth), they are prescribed a sleeping pill and told to report back. If they report no improvement, these patients may be offered CBT-I, which may not improve their insomnia because the insomnia is related to a medical condition. Thus, in all cases of insomnia, medical and psychiatric disorders need to be considered, because treating what appears to be isolated insomnia will not solve the problem.

Similarly, restless legs syndrome (RLS) can result in difficulty going to sleep, referred to as sleep onset insomnia. Patients with this condition feel an irresistible urge to move their legs and experience a creepy and crawly feeling in them, which begins or worsens in the evening. Moving the legs actually appears to improve the sensation and feeling, until this begins again. Without a proper history from the patient and questioning them about this condition, a doctor may just think that the patient has insomnia. After all, the patient may not know what to mention in their consultation with the doctor and may just report their inability to go to sleep and the resulting daytime fatigue on the following day. Reflect on Thao's story in the first part of this book. A nail technician, Thao was expected to sit for prolonged periods of time. Her symptoms became more severe and occurred earlier in the day (something called augmentation), which prompted her to present to the clinic. It was during this time that she was diagnosed with RLS and the cause for it was elucidated, which turned out to be decreased iron stores due to her menstrual cycle..

Although narcolepsy may not necessarily present as insomnia, it needs to be entertained as a cause of insomnia and restless sleep. It is the second leading cause of excessive daytime sleepiness diagnosed by sleep centers after obstructive sleep apnea but can also present as insomnia. It occurs when the nerve cells that produce orexin, a sleep-alerting agent, are depleted. The main symptoms of narcolepsy are excessive daytime sleepiness and a variety of conditions that arise from REM sleep, such as cataplexy, sleep paralysis, and hypnagogic/hypnopompic hallucinations. Cataplexy is virtually synonymous with narcolepsy, a condition in which muscle weakness is triggered by strong emotions. Patients may describe knee buckling, jaw slacking, and head dropping as just some of the weaknesses that are triggered by laughing, excitement, anger, or surprise. In narcoleptics, insomnia occurs as a result of fragmented sleep, when the individual is awakened with vivid dreams and unable to fall asleep because of the hallucinations they may experience.

As is well known, anxiety and depression can foster insomnia or be products of insomnia, acting in a bidirectional manner. Whatever the cause, it is imperative that these conditions be addressed and treated. When one sleeps poorly, this needed rest affects the brain's frontal lobe, which is necessary for attention, creativity, and executive function. In turn, not being able to pay attention, think creatively, or function adequately will fuel anxiety and perpetuate insomnia. Thus, the root of this problem needs to be addressed and treated. Insomnia is considered a risk factor for depression, as is depression for insomnia. Individuals with anxiety and depression need a consultation with a psychiatrist and/or psychologist so their symptoms can be addressed.

Chronic pain is another culprit in causing and perpetuating insomnia. The role of pain cannot be dismissed. Chronic conditions like fibromyalgia and rheumatoid arthritis, as well as acute injuries, can make it difficult to fall and stay asleep, which, in turn, decreases slow-wave sleep, a component vital for recovery. Pain creates microarousals, which are changes in a sleep state from a deeper to a lighter stage of sleep. This may lead to either a conscious or unconscious awakening. The result of both is that the brain is not obtaining the sleep it needs to be fully functional. Obviously, the treatment strategy for such insomnia is to address the underlying condition causing the pain. If it's pain in the back, for example, ibuprofen can be taken at night to minimize the awakenings, or the patient can try meditation and mindfulness. Techniques related to sleep-hygiene can also be implemented, such as 1) stopping or limiting caffeine or alcohol consumption, especially in the evening; 2) avoiding loud sounds and bright lights before bed and during the night, whether this be from television, smartphones, tablets, or computers; and 3) trying to maintain a regular sleep schedule, with anchored wake-up times.

Session 5 in Review:
What Can You Do?

What should be evident this week is the vital role that medical and psychiatric diagnoses can play in insomnia. When insomnia does not abate with sleep hygiene, sleep restriction, and cognitive therapy, one must always look to other diagnoses that hinder improvement. However, treating the other non-sleep-related diagnoses, along with the techniques we've learned so far, is the best strategy. Yes, one must focus on treating the underlying issue, but also be mindful of the various tools at our disposal. If any of the descriptions of medical conditions above sound like something you're experiencing, or if you're just experiencing persistent pain that won't go away, seek help from your family physician or internist. They're able to coordinate your care and order lab work to ensure that you don't have hyperthyroidism, for example; an overactive thyroid can cause anxiety, a rapid heart rate, and insomnia.

Session 6

Plan to Maintain Your Sleep

NOW THAT WE'RE CONCLUDING THIS 6-STEP COURSE in CBT-I, recognize that you've come a long way! Congratulations. You've learned powerful techniques, such as sleep restriction, stimulus control, and cognitive restructuring, which, I hope, have reshaped your sleep world to think about sleep in a different and more cohesive way. As you know, sleep cannot be forced, and part of this is to "let go" and allow the body to take over. Mindfulness, meditation, and guided imagery can be implemented if the rumination continues.

Look back to the stories of the individuals in the first part of this book and review how their issues were resolved. Your story may not resemble theirs exactly, but each has bits and pieces that approximates yours. Not all of the techniques will apply to your insomnia. That's fine. Hone in on those that do and learn those well. Sleep restriction will be applicable to most. Dream rehearsal will not. You'll find that, over time, these techniques will become innate. However, refrain from veering to your comfort zone. You may have to return to this book, again and again, and that's perfectly fine. Repetition of these concepts will ingrain them and make them natural. What matters is to use the arsenal at your disposal and battle the forces that have caused you those sleepless nights.

You may also want to think back to the goals you devised for yourself before this program and see the ones you accomplished. It may not be every single goal, but, surely, you did succeed at some level. Focus on the gains that you made, instead of those that you didn't. The mind has a way of focusing on failures instead of successes.

Keep an eye on your sleep efficiency. If your sleep efficiency exceeds 85%, realize that you can extend your sleep time by retiring to bed 15 minutes earlier and repeating this until you find a time that works for you. Similarly, if your sleep efficiency dwindles below 80%, recognize that you may have to retire to bed 15 minutes later. Also, acknowledge that the average amount of sleep for an adult is 7 to 8 hours, and some may even need less than this. The number of hours that you sleep is not as important as how you feel when you awaken in the morning. As with everything else, quality is more important than quantity.

If, at any point, your insomnia rears its head, review the steps that initially helped you. Are you maintaining a fixed wake-up time, with adequate sunlight to follow, as these will both strengthen your sleep drive and circadian rhythm? Is relaxation time a part of your routine? Are you using deep breathing exercises, guided imagery, and other modes to help ease your worries? Is sleep restriction still part of your routine, or are you sleeping whenever and wherever you want? Cognitively, are you worrying about things that may not even affect you or make a difference in the long term? Tackle these questions, again, because it is likely that you did not address one of these issues.

If you are taking sleep medications to fall asleep or maintain sleep, realize that you may still take these and partake in CBT-I, as long as you make a concerted effort to follow the strategies we have talked about. You may want to take half a tablet instead of one and reserve the other half as a rescue medication. Over the years, I have learned that having a "rescue" agent is just as powerful in combatting insomnia as actually taking a tablet. Knowing that something is there should you need it removes that performance anxiety we previously discussed. I have had patients who have licked their Ativan tablets and then successfully fallen asleep. This placebo effect is just as powerful as the real thing. Similarly, knowing that you have these powerful CBT-I techniques at your disposal alleviates the anxiety that prevents you from going to and maintaining sleep. You don't have to use the tools. Just realize that you have them and can refer to them if you need to.

A few final notes before we conclude our CBT-I program. Although there are tenets in this program that will serve you well, that doesn't mean that you can't experiment with them. If you read in bed, continue to do so, provided that this be for a maximum of 20 minutes. If you're unable to fall asleep because you are hungry, you can eat yogurt or other light foods (but nothing too substantial) to help satiate you for a short time. However, what must not be sacrificed is your wake-up time, which should remain anchored and stable, so that you can maintain your sleep drive. Also, be cognizant of obtaining at least 30 minutes of sunlight when you awaken, as this will keep your circadian rhythm in sync. In short, apply what you've learned, but recognize that, over time, you can adjust certain strategies that you've learned in this course to better suit your needs. Practice (in sleep) makes perfect. And continue to practice, because we're all works in progress.

Session 6 in Review: What Can You Do?

I'm hopeful that these sessions in CBT-I have served you well. Recognize the progress you have made during this time. This is just the beginning. For some, CBT-I may take some time to master, but do not revert to your old habits. Instead, review the key tenets of CBT-I—sleep restriction and cognitive restructuring—and don't forget the basic sleep hygiene techniques. The key is to let go, and not allow yourself to overthink your insomnia. Let your body, and not your mind, take over at night. It will take you where you need to go, naturally and seamlessly.

Conclusion

A T THIS POINT, I HOPE YOU'VE LEARNED THAT SLEEP is as mysterious as it is mundane. It's perplexing in so many ways, but it is also part of our daily routine, like eating, drinking, showering, and conducting our other daily activities. When we don't get enough of it, we're wrecked, but we don't die, either. In this way, we have to understand the merits of sleep without allowing ourselves to worship it, making it more special than it is. We have to be mindful of its extraordinary benefits while not allowing ourselves to be subsumed by it. To do so would allow us to be under its control when we're the ones actually in charge. Please remember that.

The individual stories in this book are also deeply important to me. I have tried to write these stories to enable you to situate yourself, as it were, in the lives and sleep conundrums of concrete characters, in the hope that it will give you a unique, empathetic perspective on how people with insomnia might think about and approach the dilemmas they face on a daily and nightly basis.

The title of this book—*Sleep Reimagined*—was chosen to convey not only how we should imagine our ideal sleep but also how to change our perception of sleep and break the cycle of insomnia. It is meant to invoke that peaceful and rejuvenating sleep you imagine for yourself after engaging in CBT-I and reading the narratives. It is a future sleep that is completely possible and within your grasp. On another level, the title refers to tools that we have at our disposal, namely visualization therapy and image rehearsal therapy, among others, where we can imagine our sleep to be what we desire. We are not powerless. We have all the tools to conquer insomnia and improve our sleep. The concept of sleep reimagined is meant to highlight this fact.

Your sleep may not improve overnight, but realize that it will improve at some point in the near future; you have all the best tools and best stories at your disposal. Don't be afraid to use them. Carpe noctem—make the night a glorious and restful one. The dark is just the night; it is not a reflection of the anxiety-ridden sleep that insomniacs have come to believe. Sleep well, readers.

Acknowledgments

THIS BOOK HAS BEEN IMAGINED (AND REIMAGINED) for quite some time. I began to develop an interest in insomnia while a fellow at the Stanford Sleep Disorders Clinic, and this fascination has persisted since.

First, an immense gratitude to my amazing literary agent, Linda Konner, who realized the great potential for this book: using case studies to illustrate how to sleep better and tackle insomnia. Without her, this book would not be possible. She championed it, and for that, I'm immensely grateful. Thank you, Linda.

Second, an enormous thanks to my fantastic editor at Countryman Press, Isabel McCarthy, who took an interest in this book from the beginning and made it come alive. Her suggestions at every stage of this book were spot-on and practical, even though I veered off topic now and again. She was the fulcrum who kept me grounded and saw this book to fruition. It was a joy to work with you, Isabel.

Other individuals at Countryman Press who assisted with the publication of this book include Ann Treistman, Jess Murphy, Devon Zahn, Allison Chi, Jessica R. Friedman, Max Winter, and countless others who remained in the background of this entire process. A big thanks to all of you.

I'm immensely grateful to my attendings at the Stanford Sleep Disorders Clinic who were instrumental in engaging me in all things sleep from my first day at the clinic. Particularly, I'd like to thank Stephen N. Brooks, Rafael Pelayo, Anstella D. Robinson, and Rachel Manber (who led the CBT-I program at Stanford). My co-fellows at Stanford, Gwynne Church and Mike Zupancic, were—and continue to be—supportive and engaging. I consider them great friends and call on them if there is a case that remains puzzling to me. Thank you, guys.

Other people who deserve mention include Nurit and Jeff Grunfeld, Avi, Josh, and Julie Handelman, Jesus and Ana Lopez, Analucia Velasquez, and Elizabeth Quinn, a close and tightly knit group with whom I had the pleasure of working at Los Angeles Sleep Institute while being the medical director there for a decade. Mona Khanna, Wendy Lori, and Walter Quigley extended their assistance at Desert Regional Medical Center in Palm Springs, California, while I was a medical director there, and I'm thankful for their friendship and assistance throughout the years.

Currently, at the Hoag Voltmer Sleep Center, I'd like to extend thanks to Yvette M. Gozzo, Marlene Grady, Elisa Popadiuk, and Jay Puangco, colleagues and staff who assist me daily and ensure that the CBT-I program at Hoag is running optimally.

At The Clinic, where I serve as a concierge sleep medicine specialist, I'd like to extend a warm thanks to Britney Blair and Tony Masri, whose support has meant a great deal.

At The Scripps Institute in San Diego, where I participated in weekly seminars during the pandemic, Derek Loewy and Steven Poceta deserve a special mention for their engaging discussions about insomnia and sleep medicine, from which I gleaned a great deal.

Although Rey Chow and Debra Di Blasi did not have a direct impact on this book, their trenchant insights and advice throughout the years have kept me grounded as a writer and scholar. I thank them immensely. You are my invisible muses.

Thanks to Lisa Lutz for encouraging me to write this unique book about sleep, a foray into non-fiction that I had never attempted. Her insights and assistance into this entire process were invaluable.

And, last, and certainly not least, are my numerous friends and family members without whom none of this would be possible. They sustained me when things become mentally draining and overwhelming, especially during the COVID-19 pandemic, when this book was written. There are too many people to name here, but you know who you are. A special thanks to Sandra Cho, Christian Gyrling, and Virgilia Virjoghe who were instrumental in brainstorming a title for this book and making it work.

This book is for the countless patients whom I've had the pleasure of knowing throughout the years and who ultimately served as the impetus for this book. I'm grateful for having learned from you. I trust that our interactions improved your sleep.

Bibliography

American Academy of Sleep Medicine. *International Classification of Sleep Disorders*. 3rd ed. Darien, IL: American Academy of Sleep Medicine, 2014.

Kabat-Zinn, Jon. *Full Catastrophe Living: Using the Wisdom of Your Body and Mind to Face Stress, Pain, and Illness*. New York: Bantam Books, 1990.

Kryger, Meir H., Thomas Roth, and William C. Dement. *Principles and Practice of Sleep Medicine*. 6th ed. Philadelphia, PA: Elsevier, 2016.

Navab, Pedram, and Christian Guilleminault. "Emerging pharmacotherapeutic agents for insomnia: a hypnotic panacea?" *Expert Opinion on Pharmacotherapy* 7, no. 13 (September 2006): 1731–38.

———. "Physiology of Sleep." In *The Child: An Encyclopedic Companion*, edited by Richard A. Shweder. Chicago, IL: University of Chicago, 2009.

Index